Little, Brown's Paperback Book Series
Little, Brown and Company
34 Beacon Street
Boston, Massachusetts 02106

Basic Medical Sciences

Boyd & Hoerl	Basic Medical Microbiology
Colton	Statistics in Medicine
Hine & Pfeiffer	Behavioral Science
Kent	General Pathology: A Programmed Test
Levine	Pharmacology
Peery & Miller	Pathology
Richardson	Basic Circulatory Physiology
Roland et al.	Atlas of Cell Biology
Selkurt	Physiology
Sidman & Sidman	Neuroanatomy: A Programmed Test
Siegel, Albers, et al.	Basic Neurochemistry
Snell	Clinical Anatomy for Medical Students
Snell	Clinical Embryology for Medical Students
Valtin	Renal Function
Watson	Basic Human Neuroanatomy

Clinical Medical Sciences

Clark & MacMahon	Preventive Medicine
Eckert	Emergency-Room Care
Grabb & Smith	Plastic Surgery
Green	Gynecology
Judge & Zuidema	Methods of Clinical Examination
Keefer & Wilkins	Medicine
MacAusland & Mayo	Orthopedics
Nardi & Zuidema	Surgery
Niswander	Obstetrics
Thompson	Primer of Clinical Radiology
Ziai	Pediatrics

Manuals and Handbooks

Alpert & Francis	Manual of Coronary Care
Arndt	Manual of Dermatologic Therapeutics
Berk et al.	Handbook of Critical Care
Children's Hospital Medical Center, Boston	Manual of Pediatric Therapeutics
Condon & Nyhus	Manual of Surgical Therapeutics
Friedman & Papper	Problem-Oriented Medical Diagnosis
Gardner & Provine	Manual of Acute Bacterial Infections
Iversen & Clawson	Manual of Acute Orthopaedic Therapeutics
Massachusetts General Hospital	Diet Manual
Massachusetts General Hospital	Manual of Nursing Procedures
Neelon & Ellis	A Syllabus of Problem-Oriented Patient Care
Papper	Manual of Medical Care of the Surgical Patient
Shader	Manual of Psychiatric Therapeutics
Spivak & Barnes	Manual of Clinical Problems in Internal Medicine Annotated with Key References
Wallach	Interpretation of Diagnostic Tests
Washington University Department of Medicine	Manual of Medical Therapeutics
Zimmerman	Techniques of Patient Care

Manual of Coronary Care

Manual of Coronary Care

Joseph S. Alpert, M.D.
Director, Samuel A. Levine Cardiac Unit, Peter Bent Brigham Hospital; Assistant Professor of Medicine, Harvard Medical School, Boston

Gary S. Francis, M.D.
Director, Coronary Care Unit and Medical Intensive Care Unit, Naval Regional Medical Center, San Diego; Instructor of Medicine, University of California, San Diego, School of Medicine, La Jolla

Foreword by Robert A. O'Rourke, M.D., Chief, Cardiology Division, and Professor of Medicine, The University of Texas Health Science Center at San Antonio Medical School

Little, Brown and Company Boston

First Edition

Library of Congress Catalog Card No. 76-47284

ISBN 0-316-03499-1

Printed in the United States of America

This book is dedicated to our parents and teachers, without whom it would never have been started; and to our wives, without whom it would never have been finished.

Foreword

Since the description of coronary care units in 1963, the number of hospitals that have opened such units has increased rapidly in the expectation that death from acute myocardial infarction would be substantially reduced. Reports from various world centers indicate a reduction in mortality of hospitalized patients with acute myocardial infarction from 30 to 20% as a result of the institution of coronary care units.

During the past ten years, the National Heart and Lung Institute has funded nine Myocardial Infarction Research Units (MIRUs) and subsequently 12 Ischemic Heart Disease Specialized Centers of Research (SCORs) in an effort to stimulate research designed to reduce morbidity and mortality in patients with coronary artery disease and, in particular, acute myocardial infarction.

In the past decade there have been numerous advances in the treatment of patients with acute myocardial infarction. These include the use of intravenous lidocaine to treat premature ventricular contractions, the development of the flow-directed balloon catheter for measuring pulmonary artery wedge pressure, and the use of various therapeutic agents to decrease myocardial oxygen demands in patients with impairment of the coronary circulation.

A practical manual for physicians, nurses, and medical technicians participating in the management of coronary care unit patients is desperately needed. This text by Drs. Alpert and Francis fulfills that need, providing important and useful information on general and specific measures used in the treatment of patients with acute myocardial infarction and its complications. The appropriate care of the acute infarction patient and its rationale are discussed from the moment the patient arrives at a medical facility through the time of subsequent outpatient rehabilitation. In addition, a suggested reading list is provided at the end of each chapter for the reader who wishes to review some subjects in greater detail. This manual provides valuable information for all medical personnel involved in the treatment of coronary care unit patients.

Robert A. O'Rourke, M.D.

Preface

This book was written in response to repeated requests from colleagues, house officers, and nurses for specific guidelines to help direct the care of patients admitted to the coronary care unit. The final product consists of 26 chapters and three appendixes that cover the entire range of coronary care. We initially began to assemble specific guidelines in protocol form, but soon found that some explanatory comments were required for each protocol. Therefore, most chapters are divided into two parts: an explanatory section followed by specific guidelines set forth in protocol fashion. The protocols are set in boldface type for easy identification. We anticipate that initially the reader will examine both the didactic and protocol sections of each chapter. Subsequently, he or she might need to refer only to the protocol sections while planning the therapeutic strategy for a particular patient. The manual should be useful in this regard to practicing physicians and house officers who could refer to it whenever faced with a difficult therapeutic decision in the coronary care unit. Nurses and paramedical personnel should find the book a concise guide to understanding the nature and direction of therapeutic endeavors in treating patients with myocardial infarctions.

The *Manual of Coronary Care* generally presents one route that we have found most effective for approaching a particular problem. We believe that for the book to be practical, such a simple, straightforward approach to each problem is best, although it will be recognized that other routes are possible. Each chapter concludes with a list of suggested readings for individuals who care to pursue the topic further.

The authors acknowledge the inspiration and assistance of the following individuals: Eugene Braunwald, M.D., Lewis Dexter, M.D., Bernard Lown, M.D., and Thomas W. Smith, M.D., of the Peter Bent

Brigham Hospital; James E. Dalen, M.D., of the University of Massachusetts Hospital; Gertrude Campbell, R.N., Eileen Edwards, Arthur D. Hagan, M.D., and W. V. R. Vieweg, M.D., of the Naval Regional Medical Center, San Diego; and Robert A. O'Rourke, M.D., of The University of Texas Health Science Center at San Antonio Medical School. We are most grateful to Lin Richter of Little, Brown and Company for her encouragement and help.

J. S. A.
G. S. F.

Contents

Manual of Coronary Care

The indications and dosages of all drugs in this *Manual* have been recommended in the medical literature and conform to the practices of the general medical community. The medications described do not necessarily have specific approval by the Food and Drug Administration for use in the diseases and dosages for which they are recommended. The package insert for each drug should be consulted for use and dosage as approved by the FDA. Because standards for usage change, it is advisable to keep abreast of revised recommendations, particularly those concerning new drugs.

1

Introduction to the CCU

Coronary Care Units (CCUs) were first organized to monitor patients with acute myocardial infarctions (MI) and to treat the lethal ventricular arrhythmias to which these patients were prone. This goal of the CCU has been generally achieved, with a consequent reduction in the acute mortality of patients with MI. The residual mortality in acute MI is related to the extent of damage that the infarcted heart sustains. Recent efforts in the field of coronary care, in addition to the understanding and treatment of arrhythmias, have been aimed at reducing the amount of myocardial necrosis in an attempt to limit left ventricular dysfunction and resultant mortality from cardiogenic shock.

Myocardial infarction results when some myocardial cells receive insufficient blood-borne nutrients and oxygen. Other myocardial cells, both adjacent to and at times remote from the center of cell necrosis, are rendered severely ischemic by the same process which caused the MI. Damage to these latter cells is not irreversible, and the focus of modern coronary care research is the delineation of therapy whereby this ischemic—but not yet necrotic—myocardium (frequently called the *border zone* or *jeopardized* myocardium) can be salvaged. Specific therapy aimed at reducing infarct size and salvaging jeopardized myocardium is discussed in Chapter 20. Most interventions that reduce the demand of myocardial cells for nutrients (especially oxygen) will be of benefit to this jeopardized ischemic myocardium. However, a reduction in myocardial oxygen demand could be detrimental if, for example, it is associated with an arterial pressure inadequate for perfusing segments of the coronary circulation distal to occlusive lesions. Thus, if the arterial diastolic pressure is reduced to 60 mm Hg or less, there may be greater myocardial ischemia despite a reduction in the myocardial oxygen demand.

Myocardial oxygen consumption has three major determinants: heart rate, myocardial contractility (the strength and vigor of myocardial contraction), and ventricular wall stress. Ventricular wall stress is related to ventricular cavity size and intraventricular pressure. Thus, both ventricular dilatation and left ventricular hypertension increase left ventricular wall stress and hence myocardial oxygen consumption. Another way of conceptualizing myocardial oxygen consumption also involves three variables: heart rate, preload or end-diastolic fiber length (directly proportional to end-diastolic left ventricular volume), and afterload or left ventricular systolic wall tension (related to left ventricular systolic pressure).

There is evidence that extensive ventricular necrosis and ischemia predispose the patient to arrhythmias and other complications of MI. The physician writing orders for a patient with an acute MI should be constantly questioning him/herself, "Is this particular order going to aid in reducing my patient's myocardial oxygen demand?"

SUGGESTED READING

Sobel, B. E. The Cardiac Care Unit: 1974. In E. Braunwald, ed., *The Myocardium: Failure and Infarction*. New York: HP Publishing Co., Inc., 1974.

Jennings, R. B., and Reimer, K. A. Salvage of ischemic myocardium. *Mod. Concepts Cardiovasc. Dis.* 43:125–130, 1974.

Maroko, P. R., and Braunwald, E. Modification of myocardial infarction size after coronary occlusion. *Ann. Intern. Med.* 79:720–733, 1973.

Sonnenblick, E. H., and Skelton, C. L. Oxygen consumption of the heart: physiological principles and clinical implications. *Mod. Concepts Cardiovasc. Dis.* 40:9–16, 1971.

2

The CCU Environment

Patients admitted to the Coronary Care Unit with an acute myocardial infarction are almost invariably distraught. The physiological concomitants of this emotional state are frequently elevated blood pressure and pulse. Increases in heart rate and left ventricular pressure result in increased myocardial oxygen demand (see Chapter 1). Increases in myocardial oxygen demand can increase myocardial ischemia and necrosis.

Considerable evidence points to a central nervous system origin for a portion of the ventricular arrhythmias associated with acute MI. This "hypothalamic" origin of ventricular arrhythmias is felt to be mediated through excessive or unopposed sympathetic nerve stimulation. In particular, ventricular arrhythmias occurring early in the course of MI are mediated via the central nervous system. It is of interest that some of these ventricular arrhythmias may be resistant to lidocaine suppression while at the same time they respond to beta blockade. (Jewitt, D. E., and Bramah, N. S. Beta blockade in acute myocardial infarction. In L. E. Meltzer and A. J. Dunning, eds., *Textbook of Coronary Care*. Philadelphia: The Charles Press, 1972.)

Experimental as well as clinical observations document the importance of psychological factors in the generation of cardiac arrhythmias. These arrhythmias may result from the combination of an unstable electrical milieu in the myocardium and centrally mediated excessive or unopposed sympathetic nerve stimulation from the emotional upset associated with admission to a CCU.

For these reasons, it is mandatory that the CCU combat the psychological trauma and the emotionally distraught state which occur in most patients with acute MI. Certain rules are axiomatic:

1. Quiet, confident, and generally serious (but not funereal) demeanor is necessary at all times in the CCU. This mental state is required of all who work in the CCU: the doctors, the nurses, the aides, the secretaries.
2. It is important to communicate to the patient (by word, by deed, and by demeanor) that everything is "under control." A careful explanation of the purpose of the various monitoring devices is invaluable in this regard. It is important to stress to the patient that the monitoring equipment is protective to him/her during the acute phase of the MI.
3. Conferences with colleagues, consultants, medical students, etc. should be held out of hearing range of the patients. Gestures or expressions that might be misunderstood by the patients should be avoided. Moreover, daily supportive contact with the patient is essential.
4. Information given to a patient's family should be straightforward but nonetheless as encouraging as possible without glossing over potential risks. (Most hospitals require that patients admitted to the CCU be placed on a seriously ill or "danger" list. The reasons for this and its implications should be explained to family members.) Physicians and nurses should try to be as positive and confident with the patient as the situation allows without being superficial or flippant.
5. Procedures that are deemed necessary (cardioversion, catheter insertion, etc.) should be explained carefully to the patient. Mention of risk should be made, but not overly dwelled on.
6. A mild sedative (e.g., diazepam) and a sleeping medication (e.g., flurazepam) are usually prescribed for patients in the CCU unless contraindicated (e.g., in chronic obstructive pulmonary disease [COPD] with CO_2 retention).
7. When patients are transferred from the CCU to another part of the hospital, the positive aspect of this transfer (i.e., the fact that the patient has re-

covered sufficiently to allow him/her to leave the CCU) should be emphasized. Patients should be warned early in the course of their CCU admission that they may be moved at any time and that this move does not represent a compromise in their care.

8. Daily contact with the outside world is important for the patient in order to prevent the development of the "ICU syndrome" (a confused and agitated state of consciousness said to be related to sensory deprivation which can occur in intensive care units). Thus, daily newspapers and visitors are encouraged; each cubicle contains a calendar and a clock; small transistor radios with earplug speakers are allowed but exciting forms of entertainment such as television are forbidden. Patients and visitors are strongly advised to refrain from stressful business and/or personal discussions and activities.

SUGGESTED READING

Hackett, T. P., and Cassem, N. H. *Coronary Care: Patient Psychology*. New York and Dallas: American Heart Association, 1975.

Cassem, N. H., and Hackett, T. P. Psychiatric consultation in a coronary care unit. *Ann. Intern. Med.* 75:9–14, 1971.

Hackett, T. P., Cassem, N. H., and Wishne, H. A. The Coronary Care Unit: an appraisal of its psychologic hazards. *N. Engl. J. Med.* 279:1365–1370, 1968.

Lown, B., Verrier, R., and Corbalan, R. Psychologic stress and threshold for repetitive ventricular response. *Science* 182:834–836, 1973.

Lown, B., Temte, J. V., Reich, P., Gaughan, C., Regestein, Q., and Hai, H. Basis for recurring ventricular fibrillation in the absence of coronary heart disease and its management. *N. Engl. J. Med.* 294:623–629, 1976.

3

The CCU Nurse

Nowhere in the hospital does the nurse have as much responsibility nor act as independently as in the CCU. Coronary care nurses should all be specially trained in the recognition and treatment of arrhythmias. They should be encouraged to "keep current" by reading, attending meetings, etc. They are constantly in the presence of the patients in the CCU, and it is the coronary care nurse who is largely responsible for creating the necessary special environment (see Chapter 2).

Some physicians (particularly early in their training) feel threatened by coronary care nurses because of the nurses' superior expertise when dealing with cardiac arrhythmias. Such feelings on the part of the physician are usually unjustified and learning to cope with them is part of his/her job. Coronary care nurses, while justifiably proud of their special abilities, are equally gracious and anxious to help physicians who are new to the CCU. This help is usually offered in an unobtrusive and hence nonthreatening manner, and physicians inexperienced in coronary care should avail themselves of the expertise of the coronary care nurse without feeling in any way diminished.

Hospitals differ in the extent to which they allow coronary care nurses freedom of action. In some institutions nurses are allowed to initiate treatment with a variety of intravenous medicines (e.g., lidocaine, atropine, morphine) according to fixed protocols. All hospitals allow coronary care nurses to defibrillate patients. House officers as well as staff physicians should know what coronary care nurses in their particular institution can and cannot do. Such an awareness prevents embarrassing, time-consuming, and divisive arguments.

It should be axiomatic in all coronary care units that physicians and nurses work together harmoniously to create the required environment (see Chapter 2).

Transfer of Patients from Emergency Area to the CCU

Potentially fatal ventricular bradyarrhythmias and tachyarrhythmias occur commonly in the early phases (first few hours) of an acute myocardial infarction (MI). Patients are commonly screened first in a triage or emergency care area. Thus, it is not uncommon for patients with acute MI to have ventricular arrhythmias during their stay in the triage or emergency area. Occasionally, patients have dangerous arrhythmias during transport from the triage or emergency area to the CCU. It is therefore important that patients be rapidly transferred to the CCU. Certain important precautions should be taken during this transfer:

Protocol

1. **A physician and a nurse (or competent, CPR-trained technician, licensed practical nurse, or aide) should accompany the patient during transfer.**
2. **The patient should be connected to a portable monitor with a clear ECG tracing visible on the screen.**
3. **The patient should have a stable IV (preferably a plastic cannula and not just a scalp vein needle) in place and running at a very slow rate. 5% D/W should be used as the infusate.**
4. **The following should accompany the patient during transfer:**
   a. **A portable battery-operated defibrillator.**
   b. **Two syringes, with needles in place, one containing 100 mg of lidocaine and the other containing 1 mg of atropine.**
5. **The patient should receive nasal oxygen from a portable oxygen tank during transfer.**
6. **A bolus of 75–100 mg of lidocaine IV prophylactically administered just before patient transfer is suggested for hospitals where there will be a significant transit time between emergency room and the CCU.**
7. **Transfer should be as rapid as is safely possible.**

8. The emergency room staff should call the CCU staff and advise them of the imminent arrival of the patient. This phone call should be made before the patient leaves the emergency room to ensure that an open bed exists.

SUGGESTED READING

Grace, W. J. *Coronary Care: Pre-hospital Care of Acute Myocardial Infarction*. New York and Dallas: American Heart Association, 1973.

5

Prognosis in Acute Myocardial Infarction

The ability to arrive at a prognosis for a particular patient with an acute infarction is not the most important skill required of the physician caring for such a patient. Indeed, signs implying a grim prognosis for a particular patient might result in a lessening of therapeutic endeavors for that individual and thus prognostication could conceivably even be counterproductive. On the other hand, the recognition of certain signs and symptoms, leading to an estimate of a patient's prognosis, enables the physician to prepare himself and the patient's family for ensuing complications.

A number of different prognostic schemes have been developed, the best known of which are detailed below:

1. Killip Classification
   Class I: no heart failure; mortality 6%.
   Class II: mild to moderate heart failure (S_3, rales no more than halfway up the back); mortality 17%.
   Class III: severe heart failure (pulmonary edema); mortality 38%.
   Class IV: cardiogenic shock; mortality 81%.
2. Peel and Norris Indices are composite scores calculated from a number of different variables (age, sex, previous history, shock, left ventricular failure, ECG, rhythm disturbances, x-ray appearance of heart size). The patient's total score is related to a specific mortality percentage with higher index scores resulting in higher predicted mortality (Appendix II gives Peel and Norris Indices).
3. Recently prognostic indices for acute MI have been derived employing invasive hemodynamic parameters obtained by means of catheterization of the pulmonary artery.

a. $\text{Prognostic index} = \dfrac{\text{DP} \times \text{MV}o_2 \text{ sat}}{\text{PCW}}$

DP = diastolic blood pressure by cuff; MVo_2 sat = pulmonary arterial blood oxygen saturation; PCW = pulmonary capillary wedge pressure. Low values for this index are associated with higher mortality. Patients in whom the index calculated equal to or greater than 250 had a mortality of only 2%. Patients with a score less than 250 had a mortality of 61%.

b. A pulmonary artery end-diastolic or PCW exceeding 28 mm Hg or a pulmonary artery end-diastolic or PCW exceeding 15 mm Hg in association with a cardiac index less than 2.3 L/min/M^2 defines a group of patients with acute MI whose mortality is 100% despite intensive medical treatment.

SUGGESTED READING

Killip, T., and Kimball, J. T. Treatment of myocardial infarction in a coronary care unit. *Am. J. Cardiol.* 20:457–464, 1967.

Peel, A. A. F., and Semple, T. Immediate prognosis in acute myocardial infarction. In L. E. Meltzer and A. J. Dunning, eds., *Textbook of Coronary Care.* Philadelphia: The Charles Press, 1972.

Verdouw, P. D., Hagemeijer, F., VanDorp, W. G., Van der Vorm, A., and Hugenholtz, P. G. Short-term survival after acute myocardial infarction predicted by hemodynamic parameters. *Circulation* 52:413–419, 1975.

Ratshin, R. A., Rackley, C. E., and Russell, R. O., Jr. Hemodynamic evaluation of left ventricular function in shock complicating myocardial infarction. *Circulation* 45:127–139, 1972.

6

The CCU Diet

Very little scientific work exists to guide the physician in selecting the best diet for a patient with an acute myocardial infarction.

Heavy meals can precipitate bouts of angina pectoris and are associated with an increase in myocardial oxygen consumption. Consequently, the CCU diet should be kept light: 1,000–1,500 cal/day.

Patients are generally kept NPO or on fluids only for a variable period of time (4–24 hours) after they first arrive in the CCU. This is done in order to observe them briefly, assuring the staff that their vital signs and clinical state are relatively stable before allowing them to eat.

Meals are usually served in small portions (six small feedings may be ideal) to diminish the possibility of increasing postprandial cardiac output.

The diet offered is soft and bland. This decreases the effort associated with eating as well as the chance of the patient's developing upsetting indigestion.

Many CCUs do not allow patients to ingest hot or cold fluids for fear that these may precipitate rhythm disturbances. Recent data do not support this contention and it is now felt that patients may ingest hot or cold fluids if desired. In addition, many CCU diets interdict the use of coffee or tea because of the fear that caffeine's sympathomimetic actions might cause arrhythmias. Patients may drink decaffeinated coffee and, if desired, weak tea, although no firm data exist to support the contention that caffeine-containing beverages actually cause disturbances in rhythm.

Many patients admitted with MI have been eating a diet rich in saturated animal fats and high in cholesterol content. A great deal of circumstantial evidence has implicated such a diet in the etiology of atherosclerosis. Most physicians feel it is prudent (although not absolutely proven effective) for post-MI patients to modify their diet by decreasing saturated fat and cholesterol intake (e.g., eggs, animal meat and fat, cream, butter) and increasing polyunsaturated fat intake (e.g., fish, chicken, vegetables, fruits).

The convalescent period following MI represents a good time to introduce the patient to his/her new diet. The CCU diet is therefore low in cholesterol and saturated fat and high in unsaturated fat.

Decreased left ventricular function with consequent decreased cardiac output can lead to sodium retention. Patients with MI should therefore not receive excessive amounts of sodium in their diet since this can lead to hypervolemia and pulmonary congestion. On the other hand, severe sodium restriction can result in hypovolemia accompanied by further depression of cardiac output, blood pressure, and urine flow. The no-added-salt diet (4–5 g NaCl in 24 hours) would seem to be a reasonable compromise.

Patients placed at bed rest and given drugs such as atropine (or drugs with atropine-like side effects) will frequently become constipated. Constipation results in straining at stool, the Valsalva maneuver, which has been shown to decrease coronary blood flow. Clearly, decreased coronary blood flow is not desirable in a patient with coronary artery disease. To combat constipation, most patients are placed on stool-softening medication on arrival in the CCU (e.g., dioctyl sodium sulfosuccinate). In addition, it seems reasonable to give average or even increased amounts of bulk in the diet of CCU patients to prevent constipation.

Some investigators feel strongly that glucose, insulin, and potassium solutions should be administered to patients with acute MI (the polarizing solution of Sodi-Pallares). Conflicting evidence exists as to whether such treatment is efficacious in preventing arrhythmias and limiting infarct size (see Chapter 20). In the absence of conclusive evidence, it seems reasonable to include healthy amounts of glucose- and potassium-containing foods in the CCU diet. This is especially true for patients who receive potassium-wasting diuretics regardless of whether they are receiving concomitant digitalis preparations or not.

In summary, a "reasonable" CCU diet is as follows:

Protocol

1. **NPO for first 4 to 6 hours after arrival in CCU. Individualize initiation of feeding according to patient's clinical status.**
2. **1,000–1,500 calorie, soft, bland, low-cholesterol and low-saturated-fat diet offered in six small feedings.**
3. **The diet should be rich in glucose, potassium, and bulk and contain approximately 4–5 g NaCl.**

SUGGESTED READING

Burch, G.E. Sick people's food. *Am. Heart J.* 85:279, 1973.

Eshleman, R., and Winston, M., eds. *American Heart Association Cookbook.* New York: David McKay Co., 1973.

7

Activity in Hospital and at Discharge from Hospital

The trend in recent years has clearly been toward earlier ambulation and discharge from the hospital of patients with acute MI. While it is conceded that pathologic studies indicate that it requires about six weeks for an infarct to be converted into a firm scar, most of the fatalities and complications occur during the first week after acute MI. In 1970 the median hospital stay in this country for acute MI was 21 days, although current data suggest that nearly 50% of patients admitted directly to a CCU with an established infarction could be discharged at seven days. The majority of patients currently stay between 12 and 21 days. Ideally, the patient is transferred from the CCU after 72 hours to an "intermediate cardiac care unit" where arrhythmia surveillance can be continued and personnel are skilled in the special needs of cardiac patients, including immediate resuscitation.

Three protocols are suggested below. Various modifications can be made in these schedules depending upon the individual case, but experience has indicated that the patient, house officers, and nurses all need some sort of definite guidelines concerning the patient's activity level following acute MI. In general, ambulation occurs on schedule unless the patient develops chest pain, postural hypotension, severe fatigue, arrhythmias, marked tachycardia, or other complications. Other variables that must be considered when individualizing the amount of activity include the emotional and physical status of the patient before the attack, associated noncardiac problems, and the response of the patient to the management. Most patients should be allowed to sit in a comfortable chair on the day after admission as long as they do not perceive fatigue. If complications do not occur, most patients are sitting up most of the fourth day and are walking on the fifth day of hospitalization. If conditions are appropriate, plans are made to go home on or about the twelfth day, and patients are permitted to walk 30 minutes in the hallway t.i.d. with supervision to prepare for this. This matter is under constant study, and it is reasonable to expect that activity levels will be stepped up even more in the future.

Protocols

12-Day Schedule

Day 1–3	**Bed rest in the CCU; may use chair in the CCU one day after admission as tolerated (e.g., 20 minutes b.i.d.).**
Day 4–6	**Bed rest in the Intermediate Cardiac Unit; may use chair most of the day; bedside commode; may be walking around the bed by day 5.**
Day 7–8	**Patient may walk to bathroom with help; transfer to ward.**
Day 9–12	**Patient may walk at will (with supervision) on the ward, may shower, and wash hair.**

14-Day Schedule

Day 1–3	**Bed rest in the CCU with bedside commode; limited chair privileges.**
Day 4–6	**Bed rest in the Intermediate Cardiac Unit; bedside commode; may sit in chair for ½ hour q.i.d. as tolerated.**
Day 7–10	**Patient may go to bathroom in wheelchair if pushed by nurse or aide; may sit in chair PRN; may begin to walk, not to exceed 1 hr/day.**
Day 11–12	**Patient transferred to ward; may walk to bathroom and elsewhere as needed, not to exceed 2 hr/day; may take a bath without washing hair.**
Day 13–14	**Patient may walk PRN and shower on the 14th day and wash hair.**

21-Day Schedule

Day 1–3	**Bed rest in the CCU with bedside commode; limited chair privileges.**

Day 4–5	**Bed rest in the Intermediate Cardiac Unit with bedside commode; limited chair privileges.**
Day 6–7	**Bed rest in the Intermediate Cardiac Unit with bedside commode; patient may sit in chair ½ hour q.i.d. or more as tolerated.**
Day 8–9	**Patient may be wheeled to bathroom by nurse or aide.**
Day 10–12	**Patient may sit in chair PRN, begin walking around bed and to bathroom.**
Day 13–15	**Patient may walk up to 2 hr/day and take tub bath.**
Day 16–21	**Patient transferred to ward and may walk PRN; may shower on the 17th day.**

SUGGESTED READING

Rose, G. Early mobilization and discharge after myocardial infarction. *Mod. Concepts Cardiovasc. Dis.* 41:59–63, 1972.

McNeer, J. F., Wallace, A. G., Wagner, G. S., Starmer, C. F., and Rosati, R. R. The course of acute myocardial infarction—feasibility of early discharge of the uncomplicated patient. *Circulation* 51:410–413, 1975.

Swan, H. J. C., Blackburn, H. W., DeSanctis, R., Frommer, P. L., Hurst, J. W., Paul, O., Rapaport, E., Wallace, A., and Weinberg, S. Duration of hospitalization in "uncomplicated completed acute myocardial infarction." *Am. J. Cardiol.* 37:413–419, 1976.

Suggested Orders in Suspected Myocardial Infarction

Many different therapeutic regimens are employed in the management of patients with acute myocardial infarction. Probably most of these programs are successful. The following set of orders constitutes a suggested program for a patient admitted to the CCU with a suspected MI. The orders themselves are written in capital letters and the comment that follows explains the purpose of that particular order.

1. ADMIT TO CCU WITH DIAGNOSIS SUSPECTED MYOCARDIAL INFARCTION. Some hospitals prefer the diagnosis to be myocardial infarction, diagnosis uncertain, or rule-out myocardial infarction. Diagnosis of myocardial infarction is discussed in Chapter 10.
2. SERIOUSLY ILL LIST (SIL). This is an administrative order which warns of the potential seriousness of the patient's condition (see Chapter 2).
3. BED/CHAIR ACTIVITY WITH COMMODE PRIVILEGES. Strict bed rest is probably not good for patients with acute MI. It can result in atrophy of normal baroreceptor function so that the patient has problems with orthostatic hypotension when he/she begins to walk. Consequently, short periods of sitting up in a chair (e.g., 20 min b.i.d.) may be allowed right from the first day of hospitalization. Patients with cardiogenic shock or severe left ventricular failure are usually not candidates for this form of early mobilization.

   Patients are frequently more comfortable and less disturbed if allowed to use a bedside commode instead of a bedpan. Activity is discussed in Chapter 7.

4. VITAL SIGNS Q 30 MIN × 4; Q 60 MIN × 2; IF STABLE, Q2H THROUGH THE FIRST 24 HR; Q4H THEREAFTER. The frequency of vital signs varies from hospital to hospital. Temperature need only be taken 2–4 times per day. Thus, most of the time, vital signs consist of respiratory rate, blood pressure, and pulse.
5. DIET: 1,500 CALORIE; LOW CHOLESTEROL, LOW SATURATED FAT, SOFT; INCREASED BULK, GLUCOSE, AND POTASSIUM. NO ADDED SALT. Diet is discussed in Chapter 6.
6. ORAL FLUID INTAKE RESTRICTED TO 1,000 ML PER 8-HOUR PERIOD. This works out to approximately 2,000 ml/day since patients have little intake during the night when they are asleep. Older CCU regimens restricted fluids more severely but recent hemodynamic data have demonstrated that most patients without overt left ventricular failure are not volume overloaded and should have a moderate fluid intake.
7. OXYGEN SUPPLEMENTATION BY NASAL PRONGS (2 L/min or more as required). Oxygen therapy is discussed in Chapter 9. Many cardiologists encourage their patients to take a deep breath every 20 minutes while awake.
8. DAILY ECGs. Since patients usually remain in the CCU for 3–4 days, 3–4 ECGs are obtained.
9. DAILY PORTABLE CHEST X-RAY. This is obtained in order to monitor pulmonary congestion secondary to left ventricular failure.
10. LABORATORY WORK
    a. DAILY (OR MORE FREQUENT) ENZYMES. Various combinations of CPK, GOT, and LDH are usually obtained. CPK is usually ordered every 4–8 hours during the first 24–36 hours of the patient's hospitalization. See Chapter 10 for a discussion of the diagnostic use of serum enzymes in MI.
    b. DAILY ELECTROLYTES. A knowledge of serum Na and K are particularly important in

patients who are receiving diuretics and digitalis preparations. Moreover, changes in cardiac output, intravenous infusion rates and diet can all influence serum electrolytes. Since electrolytes can have a major effect on cell excitability, and since patients with MI are already prone to arrhythmias secondary to altered cell excitability, it is vital to follow daily serum electrolytes until the patient's condition is stable.

c. OTHER BLOOD TESTS: CREATININE, GLUCOSE, BUN, TOTAL PROTEIN, ALBUMIN, CALCIUM, PHOSPHOROUS, CHOLESTEROL, HEMATOCRIT, WBC, ESR, PROTIME, SCREEN FOR SYPHILIS. Periodic determination of serum creatinine, glucose (daily or more often in diabetics), BUN, total protein, albumin, calcium, and phosphorous all aid in the management of acutely ill patients. These tests need not be determined every day in relatively stable patients. Serum cholesterol frequently demonstrates an early fall with MI. However, a value obtained on the first day of the patient's hospitalization frequently gives the physician a rough idea as to whether his patient is usually hyperlipidemic.

A daily hematocrit is required for patients with acute MI, since there can be a fall in this measurement during the patient's first few days in the hospital. This fall is probably related to frequent bloodletting. An occasional patient has an increase in hematocrit. The latter finding usually implies significant dehydration.

Some CCUs follow daily white blood counts and sedimentation rates as an aid in the diagnosis of MI. Both measurements show moderate elevations early in the course of acute MI. White blood counts and sedimentation rates remain elevated for approximately 1 to 2 weeks after MI (see Chapter 10). Persistently elevated values are often a sign of Dressler's syndrome (late, autoimmune pericarditis) as discussed in Chapter 19.

A rough screen of coagulation is obtained with a prothrombin time (PROTIME). A rare patient—particularly one in shock or with severe left ventricular failure—may develop disseminated intravascular coagulation (DIC) and require frequent prothrombin times as well as other tests of the integrity of the coagulation cascade. The average stable patient need have a prothrombin time determined only on admission if this value is normal.

In most states a screening test for syphilis is required on all admissions to the hospital.

11. DAILY WEIGHTS AND INTAKE (I) AND OUTPUT (O). The recording of daily weight and of intake and output is particularly important in patients with left ventricular failure.
12. 5% D/W INTRAVENOUS INFUSION (WITH BURETTE AND MINIDRIPPER) HELD AT KEEP-OPEN INFUSION RATE. A CVP line or shorter plastic cannula is the preferred type of intravenous line. Scalp vein needles are too easily dislodged and hence may become infiltrated at a critical moment.
13. MEDICATIONS
    a. LAXATIVES AND/OR STOOL SOFTENERS. Generally a daily stool softener is ordered to prevent straining at stool. See the discussion of increased bulk in the diet and its combination with stool-softening medication (see Chapter 6). Patients who are constipated despite stool softeners should be given a gentle laxative such as milk of magnesia (MOM) (usually administered h.s.).
    b. TRANQUILIZERS. Psychological factors play an important role in the genesis of arrhythmias (see Chapter 2). A mild sedative is usually prescribed q.i.d. for patients with

acute MI. Diazepam (5 mg) or chlordiazepoxide (10 mg) are the usual choices. A sleeping medication is also frequently required since patients with acute MI experience anxiety-related difficulties in falling asleep. Flurazepam (30 mg) is the sleeping medicine of choice since it tends not to disturb REM sleep patterns.

c. ANALGESICS. Propoxyphene, aspirin, and acetaminophen are effective for minor discomforts, while morphine or demerol are usually required for initial control of the pain of MI. Morphine or Dilaudid is usually preferred for pain associated with anterior or lateral infarctions while demerol is employed for inferior infarcts. The addition of morphine's parasympathomimetic actions onto the already increased vagal tone associated with inferior infarction may cause heightened vagal effects. For this reason different analgesics are used. Repeated doses of analgesics should be given every 15 to 20 minutes until pain is relieved.

d. ANTICOAGULANTS. Increasing evidence has accumulated demonstrating that small subcutaneous doses of heparin administered q8–12h prevent thrombophlebitis and associated pulmonary embolism in patients with MI. Early ambulation schedules also reduce this complication and make "minidose" heparin, if employed, necessary for only 4 to 5 days (see Chapter 21). Some cardiologists recommend the use of warfarin anticoagulants routinely in patients with MI. This is a highly controversial subject (see Chapter 21).

Protocol

1. **Admit to CCU with diagnosis: suspected myocardial infarction.**
2. **Place on SIL.**

3. **Activity: bed/chair with commode privileges.**
4. **Vital signs: q 30 min × 4; q 60 min × 2; if stable, q2h through first 24 hours and then q4h thereafter.**
5. **Diet: NPO until stable (4 to 24 hours); thereafter 1,500 calorie, low-cholesterol, no-added-salt diet (see Chapter 6).**
6. **PO fluids restricted to 1,000 cc/8 hr.**
7. **O_2 at 2 L/min by nasal prongs.**
8. **Daily ECG.**
9. **Daily portable chest x-ray.**
10. **Blood work: daily CPK (3 to 6 determinations during the first 24 hours), GOT, LDH, Na, K, Cl, CO_2, CBC, ESR. On admission and every other day: BUN, glucose, creatinine. On admission only: total protein, albumin, calcium, phosphorous, cholesterol, VDRL.**
11. **Daily weights and I and O.**
12. **IV: keep-open with 5% D/W.**
13. **Meds:**
    a. **Dioctyl sodium sulfosuccinate 100 mg PO qd.; MOM 30 cc PO hs PRN for constipation.**
    b. **Diazepam 5 mg 1 tab PO q6h.**
    c. **ASA 325 mg: 2 tabs PO q6h. PRN for headache, muscle, or joint pain. Morphine 5 mg, Dilaudid 2 mg or Demerol 75 mg (dosage is variable depending on patient's size, sensitivity to narcotics, severity of pain, relative contraindications) IV PRN for severe pain. (Usually administered by physician, but some CCUs allow nurses to administer narcotics using strict protocols.) Repeated doses to be determined by physician (repeat doses should be given every 15 to 20 minutes until pain is relieved).**

9

Arterial Blood Gases and Supplemental Oxygen Therapy

Patients with MI are usually hypoxemic. This is due in part to an intrapulmonary right-to-left shunt of desaturated venous blood. This shunt occurs because of abnormal airway (especially small airway) function in addition to ventilation-perfusion imbalances in the lungs of patients with acute MI. These pulmonary abnormalities are probably the result of increased lung interstitial water secondary to the increased left ventricular filling pressures so common in patients with MI. Another common cause of arterial hypoxemia in acute MI is chronic obstructive pulmonary disease secondary to long-standing cigarette use. Worsening hypoxemia, particularly after two to three days in the CCU, can be due to atelectasis, pneumonia, or pulmonary embolism.

Patients with MI have significant myocardial ischemia, and arterial hypoxemia probably accentuates this oxygen lack. It therefore seems reasonable to treat such patients with modest amounts of supplemental oxygen. Recent animal experiments support this view: significant reduction in experimental infarct size was obtained by means of supplemental oxygen therapy (see Chapter 20).

Protocol

1. **Patients should be placed on supplemental oxygen—2 L/min by nasal prongs, on arrival in the CCU.**
2. **Patients should have arterial blood gases determined approximately 5–10 minutes after the initiation of O_2 therapy.**

   A convenient technique for obtaining arterial blood which produces minimal discomfort is a radial artery puncture with a 22-gauge needle through a small intraepidermal wheal of 1% lidocaine. Be sure the inside of the syringe is thoroughly coated with heparin and that heparin fills the dead space of the syringe and

needle. The latter maneuver prevents air bubbles from getting into contact with the arterial blood sample.

3. **If the Po_2 in the arterial blood sample is less than 80 torr, the delivery of supplemental O_2 should be increased to 4 L/min and repeat arterial blood gases should be obtained 5–10 minutes later.**
4. **If the arterial Po_2 is still less than 80 torr, supplemental oxygen should be delivered by face mask rather than nasal prongs. In severely hypoxemic patients such as those with pulmonary edema, oxygen supplementation should be initiated by the face mask route.**
5. **Failure to obtain adequate arterial Po_2 values with face mask oxygen delivery should result in a switch to a rebreathing face mask apparatus for oxygen supplementation.**
6. **Oxygen therapy should continue at least as long as the patient is in the CCU and probably until the fourth or fifth day after infarction.**
7. **If pulmonary embolism is suspected, it may be helpful to obtain arterial blood gases while the patient is breathing room air. Oxygen therapy need be discontinued for only 7 min in patients without pulmonary disease in order to obtain a blood sample representative of room-air pulmonary function. If the patient has clinically significant obstructive pulmonary disease, it is necessary to withhold oxygen for 25 min before obtaining the arterial blood sample.**

SUGGESTED READING

Maroko, P. R., Radvany, P., Braunwald, E., and Hale, S. L. Reduction of infarct size by oxygen inhalation following acute coronary occlusion. *Circulation* 52:360–368, 1975.

Fillmore, S. J., Guimaraes, A. C., Scheidt, S. S., and Killip, T. Blood-gas changes and pulmonary hemodynamics following acute myocardial infarction. *Circulation* 45:583–591, 1971.

Biddle, T. L., Khanna, P. K., Yu, P. N., Hodges, M., and Shah, P. M. Lung water in patients with acute myocardial infarction. *Circulation* 49:115–123, 1974.

10

ECG, Enzymes, Serial Chest X-Ray Changes, and Myocardial Imaging

ECG

Medical personnel involved in the care of patients with acute MI should familiarize themselves with standard electrocardiographic textbooks which demonstrate scalar tracings of representative infarction patterns. Acute MI can be transmural or subendocardial, and the type of infarction does not necessarily relate to the complication rate or prognosis. Transmural infarctions are characterized by the evolution of Q waves and can occur in the posterior, inferior, inferolateral, lateral, anterior, apical, and anteroseptal regions of the left ventricle. Nontransmural or subendocardial infarctions are characterized by ST and T wave changes and may involve sizable amounts of myocardium or be quite small. It should be remembered that ST and T wave changes, and even Q waves can occur in the absence of any myocardial necrosis.

ENZYMES

The classic manifestations of acute MI are chest pain, serial ECG changes, and elevated serum enzymes. Specifically, the enzymes that have been used are lactic dehydrogenase (LDH), glutamic oxaloacetic transaminase (GOT), and creatinine phosphokinase (CPK). Unfortunately, as clinicians are well aware, the chest pain can be atypical, the ECG changes ambiguous, and the enzymes nonspecific. It has long been apparent that conventionally measured enzymes (LDH, GOT, CPK) are not specific for myocardial damage. It is out of this dilemma that interest in isoenzymes has developed. Isoenzymes have generally similar molecular weights and catalyze the same biochemical reactions, but have certain physical and chemical characteristics that are specific for them. The isoenzymes for LDH and CPK include fractions that are rather specific for heart muscle. LDH_1 is found primarily in extracts of heart, but all five LDH isoenzymes are also present in most human tissues. The "myocardial" LDH isoenzyme (LDH_1) is also found to a large extent in red blood cells and is particularly elevated when there is intravascular hemolysis. The cardiac isoenzyme of CPK (CPK-MB), on the contrary, is quite specific for heart muscle and is proving most useful in the diagnosis of acute MI.

One should remember that elevated serum enzyme activity reflects assay activity, not amount or concentration, and that although one assumes that this activity is released from injured tissue, peak elevation of serum enzyme activity may not correlate closely with the magnitude of tissue damage. Variables such as rate of release and clearance rate obviously play a role in determining peak activity levels, and these factors are currently not fully understood. In general, patients with peak GOT values exceeding 250 Karmen units are said to have suffered a large infarction. However, patients with large infarctions who slowly release large amounts of enzyme from the heart will exhibit peak serum values considerably lower than those seen in patients with the same extent of myocardial damage who release enzyme into the circulation more rapidly. An occasional patient with a history suggestive of acute MI will have low normal baseline enzyme values which rise over 2–3 days but never exceed the upper limits of normal for that particular enzyme. This pattern is suggestive of myocardial necrosis. The following are some general guidelines concerning the enzymes used to diagnose acute MI:

1. GOT. The activity of this enzyme exceeds the normal range within 8–12 hours after the onset of chest pain, peaks in 18–36 hours, and declines to the normal range within 3–4 days. It is rather sensitive and its failure to rise in acute MI is most

unusual. The problem is that it is elevated in a variety of disease processes, including hepatic congestion, shock, primary liver disease, and skeletal muscle disease. GOT may be increased following tachycardia when the heart rate exceeds 140 beats/min for at least 30 minutes, apparently due to associated hepatic congestion. It is commonly elevated in congestive heart failure (CHF), also secondary to hepatic congestion. SGPT (serum glutamic pyruvate transaminase) should be measured in such cases, because SGPT is more specific for liver disease, and a normal SGPT level supports the contention that elevated GOT activity is due to a nonhepatic abnormality, i.e., myocardial necrosis. GOT activity is elevated in less than 15% of patients with pericarditis, presumably reflecting subepicardial injury. Elevated GOT activity is reported in 25% to 50% of patients with angiographically proven pulmonary emboli. About 25% of patients treated with electrical cardioversion may exhibit increased GOT activity due to skeletal muscle injury. About 11% of females taking oral contraceptives will have elevated GOT, usually late in their menstrual cycle, and GOT is elevated in patients treated with clofibrate. It is also elevated following cardiac catheterization, general anesthesia, and various surgical procedures.

2. LDH. In acute MI, LDH activity exceeds the normal range within 24–48 hours, peaks in 3–6 days, and is reduced to normal in 8–14 days. Its activity is also increased by exercise and in patients with CHF, hemolysis, megaloblastic anemia, neoplasm, pulmonary embolism, shock, myocarditis, cardiac catheterization, electrical cardioversion, and inflammation. As mentioned previously, the isoenzyme, LDH_1, although more specific than LDH, has not proven particularly useful.
3. CPK. The activity of this enzyme is clearly more specific for myocardial necrosis than the other two. Typically it exceeds the normal range within

6–12 hours, reaches peak activity in 24 hours, and declines within 3–4 days to normal. Females have lower normal values. This enzyme is present in abundance in skeletal muscle, brain, and thyroid, as well as in myocardium. It probably is also present in inflammatory cells. Elevations of its activity occur with intramuscular injections, tachyarrhythmias (probably due to myocardial release), pericarditis (rarely and usually slight), myocarditis, selective coronary arteriography, severe exercise, hypothyroidism, and pulmonary embolism. As mentioned previously, the CPK isoenzyme (MB fraction) appears quite specific for myocardial damage and is the most useful enzyme test currently available for this purpose. Generally, the increase in serum CPK-MB activity parallels that of the total CPK, with elevations beginning approximately 4 hours after the onset of pain, and peaking at about 15 hours. The CPK-MB activity may peak earlier than the total CPK activity, and may decline more rapidly. Although the fractional disappearance rate of CPK from the serum varies considerably among patients, it seems to remain constant for individuals despite marked hemodynamic derangements. CPK-MB activity may be elevated following cardiac surgery in the absence of ischemic necrosis, and in patients with muscular dystrophy, perhaps due to subclinical cardiac involvement.

Since mortality following acute MI generally parallels the magnitude of peak enzyme activity, investigators have been keenly interested in using a mathematical model relating CPK activity to infarct size, both to predict the size of the infarction, and to observe the various results of interventions used to modify the infarction size (see Chapter 20). Predictions of infarct size calculated from initial serial enzyme data have now been used to monitor various interventions designed to limit infarct size. This method is not universally accepted as an accurate means of estimating infarct size, and further work is needed to validate its usefulness.

White blood counts (WBC) and erythrocyte sedimentation rates (ESR) are usually elevated in acute MI. Some hospitals employ these tests routinely in the diagnosis of MI. As a rule, the WBC varies between 12,000–15,000, but may rise as high as 15,000–20,000. There may be a modest shift to the left. Leukocytosis usually recedes after a few days and disappears by the end of a week. Persistence of the leukocytosis or very high WBCs (> 20,000) suggests the development of complications such as pulmonary embolism, pneumonia, or pericarditis. Sedimentation rates usually rise after the first few days following acute MI. The ESR may remain elevated for many weeks. Particularly high values are noted with complications such as pulmonary embolism with infarction and pericarditis.

CHEST X-RAY

Serial study of the chest x-ray in patients with acute MI is particularly helpful, especially when evaluating the temporal sequence of hemodynamic changes. One should remember that most chest films obtained in the CCU employ the portable anteroposterior technique, which tends to magnify the heart size to some extent, and makes the diagnosis of cardiomegaly less reliable. In patients with minimal or no heart failure, one may request the x-ray technician to take a six-foot posteroanterior chest x-ray with the patient sitting upright on the edge of the bed and the x-ray shot from behind.

Transudation of fluid from the pulmonary capillaries into the interstitial spaces occurs when the PCW exceeds 25 mm Hg. In fact, interstitial pulmonary edema may occur at lower wedge pressures when there has been damage to the capillary membranes resulting from hypoxia or shock. Interstitial pulmonary edema is manifested roentgenographically by Kerley "B" lines, which have been reported to occur with left atrial pressures as low as 14 mm Hg, but usually require PCWs in the 18–25 mm Hg range. Redistribution of flow to the apices, loss of the sharp marginal contour of the pulmonary vessels, development of perihilar haze, and periacinar rosette formation are other radiologic criteria of pulmonary vascular congestion and elevated PCW. Pulmonary venous distention is not a reliable index of acute cardiac failure, since chest films in patients with acute MI are not usually of a quality sufficient to evaluate pulmonary vessels.

In roughly 40% of patients with acute MI who develop pulmonary edema, there will be radiographic evidence of pulmonary congestion before rales or other clinical signs of left heart failure are present. However, in most cases, the left ventricular decompensation requires up to 12 hours to manifest itself radiographically. In the latter situation it is possible for the patient to receive immediate, successful therapy for early decompensation, only to have "roentgenographic" pulmonary edema appear after the wedge pressure has returned to normal (see McHugh et al. in Suggested Reading). This may lead to the use of potent diuretics, resulting in hypovolemia and even shock.

Additionally, a "post-therapeutic phase lag" can occur, which refers to the time required for the chest film to normalize following the treatment of elevated wedge pressure. This phenomenon is due to the time required for edema fluid to be resorbed when the wedge pressure drops with treatment. This resorption of fluid may take up to four days, and again can result in the wrong decision, i.e., continued use of potent diuretics (see Kostuk et al. and McHugh et al. in Suggested Reading). One should also be cognizant of the fact that chronic interstitial fibrosis can masquerade as interstitial edema.

MYOCARDIAL IMAGING

There has been considerable interest in recent years in the use of myocardial imaging with radionuclides to diagnose myocardial ischemia and infarction. Additionally, with the use of sophisticated and complex scintillation cameras, a *radionuclide angiocardiogram* can be obtained in the setting of acute

MI to help make a quantitative assessment of left ventricular performance. Positive scintigraphic imaging of MI has been achieved with several different radionuclides, including gallium-67 citrate, technesium-99m (Tc-99m), (SN) tetracycline, and glucoheptonate; but the most promising agent is perhaps technesium-99m (Tc-99m) stannous pyrophosphate. Positive scintigrams using this radionuclide are thought to be due to incorporation of pyrophosphate into the crystalline structure of hydroxyapatite found within damaged myocardial cells. It is believed by some that the cells must be irreversibly damaged before they will take up the phosphate. This point is somewhat unsettled, however, since diffuse and faintly positive uptake can be seen in chronically ischemic myocardium in the absence of clinical infarction, and well-localized and strongly positive scans can be seen in patients with calcified cardiac valves. Whether the faint and diffusely positive pattern seen in patients with unstable angina represents limited myocardial necrosis that is undetected by ECG and enzymes is unclear at this point.

Tc-99m stannous pyrophosphate scans become positive at 12–36 hours, remain positive up to six days after the onset of infarction, and begin to fade thereafter. They are usually negative within seven days after the onset of infarction. Most infarctions can be sharply localized by areas of increased uptake, and the procedure appears promising. Processes in which false positive images may occur include electrical cardioversion, breast tumors, functioning breast parenchyma in premenopausal females, and healing rib fractures. Of course, the radionuclide is taken up by normal bone as well. It is not clear whether acute pericarditis or infiltrative myocardial disease result in abnormal scans. Old infarctions do not appear to concentrate the radionuclide. In general, this imaging method holds promise in identifying and locating acute MI, although further experience is necessary to confirm its usefulness.

Myocardial perfusion imaging with tracers that

concentrate in myocardial cells in proportion to blood flow also has diagnostic usefulness in acute MI. Thallium[201], cesium, rubidium and potassium[43] have been used for this purpose, although thallium appears to accumulate in the normal myocardium to a greater degree and has relatively low energy radiation that is more suitable for imaging. It does not clearly distinguish between acute infarction and ischemia, however, and cannot differentiate old and new infarctions.

Protocol

1. **Enzymes should be ordered at least daily for the first three days of the patient's hospitalization. More frequent enzyme analysis may be ordered on the first day (particularly for CPK).**
2. **A portable chest x-ray should be ordered at least daily for the first three days of the patient's hospitalization. Additional chest films should be obtained if the patient's clinical condition alters, i.e., pulmonary edema, hypotension, etc.**
3. **Radionuclide myocardial imaging may be a useful adjunct in the diagnosis of acute MI. Its eventual usefulness in the CCU remains to be determined.**

SUGGESTED READING

Roberts, R., and Sobel, B. E. CPK isoenzymes in evaluation of myocardial ischemic injury. *Hosp. Practice* 55–62, Jan, 1976.

Sobel, B. E., and Shell, W. E. Serum enzyme determinations in the diagnosis and assessment of myocardial infarction. *Circulation* 45:471–482, 1972.

Parkey, R. W., Bonte, F. J., Meyer, S. L., Atkins, J. M., Curry, G. L., Stokely, E. M., and Willerson, J. T. A new method of radionuclide imaging of acute myocardial infarction in humans. *Circulation* 50:540–546, 1974.

Kostuk, W., Barr, J. W., Simon, A. L., and Ross, J. Jr. Correlations between the chest film and hemodynamics in acute myocardial infarction. *Circulation* 48:624–632, 1973.

McHugh, T. J., Forrester, J. S., Adler, L., Zion, D., and Swan, H. J. C. Pulmonary vascular congestion in acute myocardial infarction: hemodynamics and radiologic correlations. *Ann. Intern. Med.* 76:29–33, 1972.

11

Arrhythmias and Their Treatment

All major forms of arrhythmias occur in the acutely ischemic myocardium, and standard textbooks should be employed to develop a fundamental understanding of the anatomy of the conduction system and the electrophysiologic principles of arrhythmias. Excellent examples of all the arrhythmias discussed in this chapter can be found in Marriott's and Constant's books on electrocardiography (see Suggested Reading). The following is an abbreviated approach to common rhythm disturbances in the setting of acute MI.

SINUS BRADYCARDIA

This is a sinus mechanism with a ventricular rate of less than 60 beats/min. It is a frequent accompaniment of acute MI, particularly in the early phase of inferior infarction. There has been considerable recent investigation and debate as to whether this rhythm affords a "protective" effect by raising ventricular fibrillation threshold. Although this controversy has not yet been completely resolved, the final decision to treat sinus bradycardia must be based on the clinical judgment of the physician. In the absence of symptoms, and when there are signs of good systemic perfusion, adequate blood pressure, and no significant ventricular irritability (automaticity), careful observation may be all that is required. If the rate consistently drops below 50, or if the patient has signs of hypoperfusion, including chest pain, frequent PVCs or low blood pressure, treatment should be instituted with intravenous atropine (an agent with vagolytic properties) provided no contraindications are present. The drug should be given by bolus in doses of 0.6–1 mg. Intravenous atropine in doses of 0.5 mg or less may paradoxically slow the heart by enhancing central nervous system parasympathetic outflow. If the heart rate does not increase in 2–4 minutes, the dose should be repeated. Should symptomatic bradycardia still persist, a temporary pacemaker would be preferable to other positive chronotropic measures such as an isoproterenol infusion, because pacing results in less oxygen demand (chronotropic = affecting the time or rate, i.e., heart rate). If atropine is initially successful, further doses should be repeated only if necessary, since repeated atropine usage may result in intolerable side effects such as ileus, glaucomic crisis, urinary obstruction, and, particularly in older patients, bizarre mental behavior. If the drug has to be used on more than three repeated occasions (such as q 2–4 h), careful consideration should be given to the alternative treatment, pacing.

SINUS TACHYCARDIA

This is a sinus mechanism with a ventricular rate greater than 100 beats/min. The upper limit of the rate is vague and varies according to age and physical condition, but in adults is usually considered to be 150 beats/min. This is an extremely important arrhythmia in the CCU and can carry an ominous prognosis, since myocardial oxygen consumption (MVo_2) is linearly related to heart rate, and infarct size is related to MVo_2 (see Chapters 1 and 20). This rhythm disturbance should be aggressively investigated to see if there is some treatable extracardiac or cardiac cause, such as residual chest pain, infection, anxiety, pericarditis, CHF, or even the discomfort associated with fecal impaction. If there is no obvious explanation for the tachycardia, and the patient appears adequately sedated, it may be assumed that the elevated rate is on the basis of hypovolemia or extensive MI. This latter differential can be extremely difficult, even for the seasoned clinician, and it may be important to resolve the issue at once since hypovolemia is correctable and sinus tachycardia due to extensive myocardial necrosis implies a poor prognosis. If the rate is greater than

100–120 and the volume status is unclear, one should measure left-sided filling pressures with a flow-directed catheter. Monitoring the central venous pressure (CVP) is frequently not a useful exercise in this setting, since right atrial pressure may be low despite elevated left atrial pressure, in which case additional volume might precipitate pulmonary edema. Moreover, the CVP may be elevated in patients with cor pulmonale secondary to chronic obstructive pulmonary disease (COPD) in whom left-sided filling pressures are usually low and in whom the addition of a potent diuretic could provoke hypotension. If the left-sided pressures are found to be low (< 10 mm Hg), adding volume to raise the pulmonary capillary wedge pressure to 15–18 mm Hg will frequently correct the hypovolemia and the sinus tachycardia. If left-sided filling (wedge) pressures are elevated (> 18 mm Hg), diuretic therapy may be useful. Remember that both hypervolemia (elevated filling pressures) and hypovolemia (low filling pressures) can increase MVo_2 and cause sinus tachycardia. These are unfavorable situations that can often be corrected, but the wrong choice of treatment (volume expansion vs diuretics) can provoke catastrophe (see also Chapters 13 and 15).

Occasionally a small dose of propranolol is employed to slow sinus tachycardia, provided left-sided filling pressures are being monitored and there is no evidence of CHF (i.e., normal PA saturation, PCW less than 18 mm Hg) or other contraindications. One to three mg may be given slowly IV every 2–3 hours. Obviously this is not conventional therapy and further investigation of the use of adrenergic beta blockade in acute MI is currently underway. The ideal candidate for this form of therapy is the individual whose sinus tachycardia is the result of persistent agitation rather than left ventricular failure or hypovolemia.

ATRIAL FIBRILLATION (AF)

This arrhythmia is said to occur in 10% of patients with acute MI. It may be present on admission or may occur during the course of the acute infarction. It exacts two hemodynamic penalties: loss of the atrial transport mechanism and rapid heart rate with decreased diastolic filling period. It may be well tolerated, or it may result in catastrophic impairment. Obvious noncardiac causes should be looked for and corrected if possible: electrolyte disturbances, hypoxia, pulmonary embolism, or thyrotoxicosis. Occasionally atrial infarction or pericarditis will cause AF. Treatment of this arrhythmia depends on ventricular rate and hemodynamic status. Rarely, a slow ventricular response occurs, resulting in symptoms or signs of hypoperfusion. This should be treated with a pacemaker, and digitalis should be withheld if previously given. Usually, the ventricular response is rapid (> 140) and there may be deterioration (pulmonary edema, hypotension, etc.). In this situation cardioversion is indicated. Cardioversion should be performed following the administration of intravenous diazepam (Chapter 22). It is probably best to begin with 100–200 watt/sec, since AF is rarely reverted with less energy. It should be remembered that hypokalemia must be corrected, and lidocaine should be given just prior to cardioversion if the patient has been on digitalis (see Chapter 22).

When the ventricular rate is between 90 and 140 and the patient is otherwise stable, increments of intravenous digoxin (0.25 mg) should be given every 3–4 hours to slow the ventricular response to optimal levels (70–80). Small doses of propranolol (10 mg PO q.i.d.) may also be employed to slow the ventricular response in AF. If the rate remains persistently elevated despite several doses of digitalis, cardioversion should be considered, since a rapid ventricular response results in increased myocardial oxygen consumption. Once the ventricular rate stabilizes, or if the patient presents with an optimal ventricular response, maintenance oral digoxin (0.25 mg per day) may be instituted, provided renal function is adequate. It is not necessary to attempt cardioversion if the rate is optimal and the patient is stable. Cardioversion may be done electively prior to discharge, or the patient may be left in AF if this is clinically appropriate (see Chapter 22). If the decision is made to cardiovert the patient, it is probably wise to institute antiarrhythmic therapy (e.g., quinidine, procainamide) prior to the procedure, since sinus rhythm is more likely to persist if the cardioversion is successful. In addition, if the procedure is successful, antiarrhythmic therapy should be maintained after cardioversion (see Chapter 22).

ATRIAL FLUTTER

This condition typically results in an atrial rate of between 280 and 320 beats/min with a 2:1 AV conduction ratio and a ventricular rate of about 150. It is occasionally seen in the setting of acute MI (about 6%). Because of the rapid ventricular rate, cardioversion is the treatment of choice. The protocol for cardioversion is given in Chapter 22: antiarrhythmic therapy is instituted prior to and following cardioversion. Usually this arrhythmia is responsive to 25–50 watt/sec. When digitalis is used to treat it, heroic doses are frequently required, time is lost, and cardioversion may still have to be resorted to later, often at greater risk due to previously administered digitalis.

PAROXYSMAL ATRIAL TACHYCARDIA (PAT)

This arrhythmia may rarely provoke or complicate acute MI. The rhythm is a regular supraventricular tachycardia with a rate between 160 and 300 (usually about 180) beats/min. The ventricular response in PAT is usually faster than in sinus tachycardia and atrial flutter with block and can be distinguished from ventricular tachycardia by its narrow QRS (unless there is associated aberrancy or bundle-branch block). Sustained PAT should be terminated immediately, even if there is no hemodynamic compromise, because the excessive heart rate leads to marked increases in MVo_2. Carotid massage should be attempted, and if this is unsuccessful, cardioversion is indicated. Usually 25 to 50 watt/sec will restore sinus rhythm. Termination of this arrhythmia with pressor agents, Valsalva maneuvers, and edrophonium is to be avoided in the setting of acute MI. Antiarrhythmic therapy with agents such as digoxin and quinidine sulfate is useful for maintaining the patient in sinus rhythm. Brief and recurrent episodes of PAT should be treated with digoxin and at times quinidine.

PREMATURE ATRIAL CONTRACTIONS (PACs)

These rhythms are common in acute MI. The P waves have a different configuration from normal, and may be peaked or inverted. They occur prematurely and result in an irregular rhythm. They are usually followed by a normal QRS, but may not always conduct through to the ventricle (blocked PACs), particularly when they occur in the refractory period of the preceding QRS. They are frequently the result of CHF, hypoxia, or electrolyte disturbance and generally require no treatment. PACs are not infrequently the harbinger of atrial fibrillation.

WANDERING ATRIAL PACEMAKER

This is due to P-waves of varying ectopic origin (and of varying shape and position) resulting in a somewhat irregular rate. This arrhythmia should be approached in a manner similar to that for PACs.

PAT WITH BLOCK

This arrhythmia is unusual in the CCU. It is characterized by an atrial rate of 150–240, and usually results in a ventricular rate of about 110–120. The P waves are frequently smaller than usual and sometimes change shape. The differential diagnosis is usually between this rare arrhythmia and atrial flutter. Atrial flutter usually has larger P-waves (frequently "saw-toothed") and a faster ventricular rate (150). PAT with block is commonly due to digitalis toxicity. In this setting, digitalis should be withheld and potassium salts administered, even if the serum potassium is normal. Cardioversion is contraindicated in PAT with block from digitalis toxicity.

JUNCTIONAL RHYTHMS

These are said to occur in 3% to 16% of patients with acute MI. A recent report indicated that the incidence may be as high as 40% if computer-assisted continuous magnetic-tape recordings are used for detection. This arrhythmia originates within the bundle of His (the atrioventricular (AV) node has no pacemaking cells). The QRS complex is of normal duration, resembling the patient's normally conducted sinus beats. This rhythm may be slower than the normal sinus rate, in the range of 40–60 beats/min, in which case it is a protective escape rhythm of no primary significance and should not be suppressed. If the ventricular response is extremely slow or clinical deterioration occurs, consider atropine and/or pacemaker therapy. Occasionally nodal beats occur as "extra systoles," but they need not be as aggressively abolished as in the case of ventricular premature beats. Digitalis excess, CHF, hypokalemia, and hypoxia should be considered as possible etiologies and corrected if present. Occasionally, junctional rhythms may begin abruptly with rates of 70–130 beats/min (accelerated junctional rhythm). Such rhythm disturbances resemble supraventricular tachycardias such as PAT, and if simple maneuvers such as carotid massage do not abort the disturbance, cardioversion with low-watt energy levels should be considered when the rate is rapid (heart rate > 120 beats/min). Again, digitalis toxicity should be considered, and hypokalemia should be corrected.

MULTIFOCAL ATRIAL TACHYCARDIA (MAT)

This rhythm is also known as chaotic atrial tachycardia and is not infrequently found in very seriously ill elderly patients, particularly when there is associated chronic obstructive pulmonary disease (COPD). It frequently carries a poor prognosis. The ventricular rate may vary between 50 and 150 beats/min. The atrial (and ventricular) rhythm is irregular due to varying P-R intervals and varying degrees of AV block. The P waves vary in configuration with at least two ectopic foci. The P waves are often peaked and tent-shaped, and the atrial rate may be extremely rapid, sometimes 250 beats/min. MAT may resemble ventricular tachycardia if there is associated QRS aberration or bundle-branch block. Multifocal atrial tachycardia is refractory to the usual treatment for supraventricular arrhythmias, and therapy directed to the underlying disease is more important than the administration of antiarrhythmic drugs. CHF, COPD, and electrolyte imbalance should be corrected. Cardioversion entails some risk and is generally not successful.

AV DISSOCIATION

This term refers to a group of arrhythmias in which the atria and ventricles beat independently, so that the P waves and the QRS complexes have no certain relationship. This condition is seen in complete AV block, ventricular tachycardia, and various supraventricular arrhythmias. The treatment obviously depends on the underlying cardiac mechanism, the ventricular rate, and the patient's condition.

PREMATURE VENTRICULAR CONTRACTIONS (PVCs)

Also called ventricular premature beats, these are omnipresent in patients who have sustained an acute MI and frequently predict the onset of more serious ventricular arrhythmias. They are characterized by widened, bizarre QRSs with abnormal appearing T waves occurring early in the cardiac cycle without any meaningful relationship to the preceding P wave. Ventricular escape beats and rhythms which occur in the setting of AV block should be considered separately. In coronary care units with continuous monitoring, PVCs have been noticed in almost all patients with acute MI if their rhythm is recorded for at least 24 hours. Empirically, a PVC frequency greater than 5 beats/min is considered potentially dangerous, and antiarrhythmic therapy is recommended. It is believed by many that this now-universal approach is responsible for the apparent reduction in acute MI mortality noted in CCUs during the 1960s. Physiologists and clinicians have also long been aware that the coupling interval between the preceding beat and the PVC, i.e., the degree of PVC prematurity, has arrhythmogenic significance. When the R wave of the PVC falls on the T wave of the preceding beat, ventricular tachycardia or fibrillation may be provoked. This "R on T" phenomenon is considered an indication for antiarrhythmic therapy. However, recent studies have indicated that the malignancy of a ventricular ectopic beat may not necessarily be determined by its coupling interval or its configuration. Ventricular bigeminy, and PVCs occurring in couplets (pairs) are also indications for immediate antiarrhythmic therapy in the setting of acute MI.

It is important, of course, to remember that PVCs in the presence of acute MI may not always be due to ischemia. Hypokalemia and CHF can provoke ventricular irritability and must be corrected. Attention should be paid to anxiety and hypoxemia. Occasionally, CVP lines or a Swan-Ganz catheter will provoke PVCs and atrial arrhythmias. The PVCs usually take the configuration of a left bundle-branch block in these cases, since they are generated from the right ventricle. This situation is usually easily corrected by repositioning the catheter.

Lidocaine administered intravenously is probably

the most widely used agent for the treatment of cardiac arrhythmias following acute MI. It is clearly the treatment of choice for ventricular irritability in the presence of acute MI. Allergic reactions to the drug are almost unknown and it has a wide margin of safety. Historical information from the patient about an allergy to procaine employed by the dentist can usually be ignored, since there is no cross reactivity between procaine and lidocaine, and to withhold the agent in a life-threatening arrhythmia would be considered poor judgment. If there is any serious question, a scratch test can be done on the skin. Some authorities advocate the use of lidocaine prophylactically for all patients with acute MI, but most CCUs employ it only for the indications mentioned above. In patients with presumed normal cardiac output and hepatic function, an initial bolus of 1.5 mg/kg (100 mg in a 70 kg person) is given over several minutes (very rapid injections may lead to transient toxic side effects), followed by a 2 mg/min continuous infusion drip. In patients with CHF or known mild hepatic impairment, a bolus of 75 mg is given followed by a 1.5 mg/min drip. In patients with markedly reduced cardiac output or shock, 0.75 mg/kg (about 50 mg) is given in a bolus followed by a 0.7–1 mg/min drip. The half-life of lidocaine is approximately 2 hours. If the infusion rate needs to be increased from 2 mg/min to 3 mg/min, an additional bolus injection of 25 mg is given intravenously. Because of the marked fat solubility of the drug, simply increasing the continuous infusion rate would require several hours to reach a new steady-state level. Likewise, when a decision is made to discontinue lidocaine, weaning is not necessary; simply stopping the infusion will suffice. Patients with PVCs resistant to lidocaine are not rare, but other causes (such as infiltrated IVs) should be sought before using the maximal continuous infusion rate of 4 mg/min.

Lidocaine is metabolized in the liver, and agents which induce hepatic enzymes, such as phenobarbital, may increase lidocaine metabolism, while drugs such as isoniazid and chloramphenicol (which may depress hepatic function) may decrease lidocaine metabolism. Serious toxic side effects include focal and grand mal seizures, psychosis and, rarely, respiratory arrest. Paresthesias, muscle twitching, disorientation, drowsiness, and reduced hearing may occur and may necessitate reducing or stopping the drug. Convulsions respond to intravenous diazepam or barbiturates, and, frequently, stopping the infusion will ameliorate the seizure. Lidocaine appears to have minimal negative inotropic effects (inotropic = affecting the force or energy of contraction), and heart rate, blood pressure, and cardiac output do not significantly change unless very large doses are given. Additionally, the drug has little or no effect on the conduction system and can be used safely in the presence of conduction disturbances.The threshold response to artificial pacing is not changed by lidocaine. The therapeutic plasma level varies from 1.4 to 6 μg/ml.

Intravenous procainamide is also effective against PVCs in acute MI, and it is a relatively safe alternative to lidocaine. It can be employed together with lidocaine to suppress ventricular ectopic activity refractory to either drug alone. Procainamide should be given intravenously by injection 50–100 mg every 5 min until the arrhythmia is abolished, a total of 1 g of the drug has been given, or untoward side effects appear (e.g., hypotension or gross widening of the QRS interval). A loading dose need not be given, and if a continuous infusion is required, the usual rate is 2 mg/min. The effective plasma concentration using intravenous procainamide is 4–8 μg/ml, which appears to result in no significant alteration in hemodynamic function. The drug causes minimal prolongation of AV conduction time but significant prolongation of His-Purkinje conduction time and should therefore be used with caution in patients with impaired conduction systems (bundle-branch block or ventricular conduction delay) unless an artificial pacemaker is in place. The drug can also increase the threshold response to artificial pacing and may result in failure of the pacemaker to initiate a ventricular depolarization.

It has been suggested that lidocaine is more effective than procainamide in preventing ventricular reentrant activity induced by early premature beats. Re-entry is characterized by closely coupled beats with fixed coupling intervals and results from depressed conductivity in an ischemic area of the ventricle. PVCs due to increased automaticity of the Purkinje tissue of the ventricle appear to be less likely to provoke ventricular tachycardia and fibrillation. The distinction between the two mechanisms is not always clear on the scalar tracing. Despite similarities in the electrophysiological properties of certain antiarrhythmic drugs, it is possible for ventricular irritability which cannot be suppressed by one antiarrhythmic agent (i.e., procainamide) to be suppressed by another antiarrhythmic drug which has the same electrophysiological properties (i.e., quinidine). The plasma half-life of procainamide is about 3½ hours, and the drug should be stopped if the QRS prolongs by more than 50%. The kidneys are responsible for most of its elimination and the half-life is prolonged when there is renal impairment. Frequently, the drug is poorly tolerated when administered for prolonged periods.

Occasionally diphenylhydantoin (DPH) is useful for suppressing PVCs associated with acute MI, particularly when there is concomitant digitalis intoxication. Its mechanism of action is probably most similar to lidocaine, and in the acute situation the recommended dose is 50–100 mg IV every 5 min until toxicity occurs, the arrhythmia is controlled, or 1,000 mg of DPH has been given. Following the initial loading dose, a 500 mg dose should be given in 24 hours, and the patient should then be started on maintenance therapy consisting of 300–400 mg once daily. The mean plasma half-life is 22 hours and hepatic dysfunction may result in toxic blood levels. Plasma concentrations between 10 and 18 μg/ml are therapeutic. Many drugs interfere with the pharmokinetics of DPH, and side effects such as hypotension, ventricular fibrillation, and asystole make it a less-than-optimal antiarrhythmic agent. Additionally, the chronic oral administration of DPH produces countless untoward effects that make it undesirable for prolonged use. The drug has a variable effect on the conduction system but usually promotes AV conduction and has little effect on the His-Purkinje system. DPH generally has no significant clinical hemodynamic effect but may rarely depress left ventricular function.

Quinidine sulfate may also be used to suppress PVCs accompanying acute MI, although it is more commonly preferred for long-term suppression of arrhythmias. Part of the reason for this is that the drug has a poor margin of safety when given parenterally, and many authors suggest that it be given only orally. Hypotension is the main drawback to its parenteral use, and shock unresponsive to sympathomimetic agents has been reported in dogs. The mechanism of action of quinidine is similar to procainamide. The half-life varies considerably from patient to patient, but averages about 7 hours. The usual dose is 1–2.4 g/24 hr in divided doses given at 6 hr intervals. Therapeutic plasma levels average 2.3–5 μg/ml using the double extraction method but are higher using precipitation assays. The drug is metabolized in the liver, and patients with hepatic dysfunction are more likely to exhibit toxicity, even at levels ordinarily considered nontoxic (due to loss of protein binding). Patients who are anephric or have poor renal function may paradoxically need more frequent doses, and plasma level measurements are recommended. The drug has little intrinsic myocardial depressant activity in therapeutic doses, but the conduction system is clearly affected. Quinidine shortens AV conduction time (probably via vagolytic action) and prolongs His-Purkinje time, and caution is indicated when the drug is used in the face of an already jeopardized conduction system. Mild nausea, diarrhea, and tinnitus frequently occur and are not necessarily reasons for stopping the medication if these side effects are transient or easily controlled with antiemetic or antidiarrheal drugs.

When conventional agents have failed and no contraindications (e.g., LV failure, bronchospasm, heart block, bradyarrhythmias) exist, propranolol should be considered for the suppression of ventricular ectopy in acute MI. A pulmonary artery catheter is useful for monitoring left-sided filling pressures when employing this agent. If the PCW is >18 mm Hg, the drug should not be used, or should be stopped if already in use. The maximum dose is 0.15 mg/kg (up to 10.5 mg for a 70 kg person) given intravenously at a rate not exceeding 1 mg/min with careful monitoring of the blood pressure, electrocardiogram, and wedge pressure. Frequently only 2–3 mg are necessary, and this dose may be repeated every 6 hours, or more frequently if ectopy recurs. The patient may be placed on oral maintenance therapy, the dose of which varies considerably, but usually is at least 80 mg/day (20 mg q.i.d.). The liver metabolizes propranolol, which has a half-life of 3–4.6 hr. Therapeutic plasma levels range from 40 to 85 ng/ml. Myocardial depression is the drug's most well-known untoward effect; others include conduction disturbances, bradycardia, fatigue, bronchospasm, and unrecognized hypoglycemia, all of which can be extremely detrimental in the setting of acute MI. The drug, in addition to slowing sinus node discharge, slows AV nodal conduction but has no effect on the His-ventricular (H-v) interval. Propranolol may be useful in early acute MI (when sympathetic overdrive may be responsible for most of the ectopy) and in digitalis toxicity. Rapid withdrawal of the drug may provoke angina pectoris and MI (see Chapter 25).

Occasionally PVCs may occur with acute MI due to the mechanism of *parasystole*. This mechanism is identified by varying coupling intervals in which the interectopic intervals are equal to a multiple of the shortest interectopic interval. Long rhythm strips are sometimes needed to make this diagnosis. The arrhythmia usually arises from an independent ventricular pacemaker and does not ordinarily deteriorate into sustained ventricular tachyarrhythmias. It responds less well to antiarrhythmic therapy, and aggressive treatment may lead to lidocaine toxicity. In fact, treatment of this arrhythmia may be unnecessary.

VENTRICULAR TACHYCARDIA (VT)

This arrhythmia is conventionally described as a sequence of three or more ventricular extrasystoles at rates ranging from 100 to 250/min. It has been described as a "disorder which is simple to terminate, only rarely difficult to prevent, but invariably impossible to diagnose with certainty." It is frequently seen during acute MI (16–40%) and its occurrence is favored by large infarctions and CHF. The mechanism of ventricular tachycardia has long been ascribed to an accelerated discharge from a single ventricular ectopic focus, but recent evidence suggests that many episodes of VT with acute MI are due to re-entry. When the rate of VT is less than 100 (this figure being used somewhat arbitrarily), the rhythm is usually considered *accelerated idioventricular rhythm* and takes on a different connotation; when the rate exceeds 250 beats/min, it is best to consider the rhythm *ventricular flutter.* Most episodes of VT have considerable regularity, with minimal beat-to-beat variation. There is more irregularity when the arrhythmia begins or is terminated, and variation in regularity is also more common in accelerated idioventricular rhythm (see below). Cardiac function is usually compromised, although beats generated from the apex of the left ventricle may be more hemodynamically effective than beats arising from basilar areas. Any sign of AV dissociation such as fusion due to capture beats is of diagnostic aid in identifying VT. AV dissociation can result in wide splitting of the first and second heart sounds, variable intensity of the first heart sound, and intermittent cannon "a" waves in the jugular pulse. Carotid sinus massage is ineffective in slowing the ventricular rate. The diagnosis of VT is further supported when the QRS complexes have a morphology similar to the patient's preexisting PVCs. Diagnostic maneuvers should not delay treatment for this life-threatening arrhythmia. If the patient is unconscious or in shock a thump to the precordium followed by electrical cardioversion (when sinus rhythm is not restored) is recommended. Frequently only 10 watt/sec will restore normal sinus rhythm. However, if this is not successful, energy levels of 50 or 100 watt/sec should be employed. If the patient is otherwise stable, a brief trial of an antiarrhythmic agent is warranted as a first approach. An intravenous bolus of 50–100 mg of lidocaine should be given, and if the tachyarrhythmia is not abolished in 2 min, a repeat dose of 50 mg should be given. If the rhythm disturbance persists, electrical cardioversion should be performed. Whether one gives analgesia depends on the seriousness of the clinical situation. If the patient is alert and needs sedation, diazepam should be given (at least three 5 mg IV doses at 2-min intervals) until the patient is lightly asleep. It is standard practice to begin a lidocaine drip at 2 mg/min once VT has been abolished and sinus rhythm has been restored. This should be started following a loading dose of lidocaine and should be infused prophylactically over the succeeding 24 hours. Recurrent VT or breakthrough PVCs should be managed as described previously in the section on PVCs.

ACCELERATED IDIOVENTRICULAR RHYTHM (AIVR)

This is an interesting and somewhat controversial arrhythmia known by a wide variety of names (frequently referred to incorrectly as "slow ventricular tachycardia"). Although it is seen in many different heart conditions, as well as in cases of digitalis intoxication, it is not rare (13–30%) during the first 48 hours of acute MI, particularly in inferior MIs. It is characterized by three or more widened QRS complexes occurring at a rate similar to the prevailing sinus rate and may alternate with periods of sinus rhythm. The first beat of a paroxysm tends to occur during the slow phase of sinus arrhythmia and has a long coupling interval to the preceding beat. It nearly always occurs at a rate of less than 100 and should not technically be considered a "tachycardia." Dissociated P waves can be seen in the majority of cases of AIVR, and the beats are not preceded by His deflections on His bundle electrograms. This confirms the supposition that AIVR is not supraventricular in origin.

A benign course has been observed in cases of AIVR, and the usual teaching has been not to suppress these beats if the patient is otherwise stable. In fact, some authors believe that treatment may be contraindicated, since suppression of what may be an "escape" mechanism can result in asystole. However, other authorities believe the arrhythmia is due to an ectopic focus with intermittent exit block. If the arrhythmia results in a slow ventricular rate with attendant problems such as hypotension or other signs of hypoperfusion (which can in part be due to loss of "atrial kick"), then treatment with atropine 0.8–1.0 mg IV is recommended provided there are no contraindications. Atropine increases the sinus rate, thus overdriving the ectopic focus. If atropine is contraindicated or fails to abolish the rhythm, an artificial transvenous pacemaker should be considered. Some authors advise the use of lidocaine to abolish this arrhythmia. This agent may be useful in AIVR; a recent report documented the fact that 83% of patients with this arrhythmia also displayed paroxysmal (rapid) ventricular tachycardia occurring in a rather unpredictable manner. (deSoyza, N., Bissett, J. K., Kane, J. J., Murphy, M. L., and Doherty, J. E. Association of accelerated idioventricular rhythm and paroxysmal ventricular tachycardia in acute myocardial infarction. *Am. J. Cardiol.* 34:667–670, 1974.) Currently, the treatment of AIVR remains controversial and rests in large part on the physician's judgment.

BIDIRECTIONAL VENTRICULAR TACHYCARDIA

This is an uncommon arrhythmia characterized by QRS complexes with a right bundle-branch block pattern in the frontal plane with an alternating morphology (seen only in the limb leads): an upward complex in one beat and a downward complex in the next. The rate is between 140 and 180 in most cases; the QRS is widened, with an axis in the frontal plane alternating between −60 to −80 degrees and +120 degrees. Bidirectional VT is most often seen in the setting of digitalis intoxication but can occur in acute MI. The ectopic focus is probably ventricular, as the complexes are not preceded by a His spike during His electrograms. The rhythm can be abolished with intravenous lidocaine.

VENTRICULAR FIBRILLATION (VF)

This arrhythmia is easily recognized by its chaotic, undulating morphology which is due to wandering of the cardiac impulse continuously along constantly changing pathways. This results in fully contracting fibers and fully relaxed fibers at the same time. When it occurs in an organized, coarse fashion, it may spontaneously revert to a less primitive rhythm, but this is rare, and immediate cardioversion is always indicated. When a patient is found pulseless, even when the nature of the arrhythmia is not clear, so-called blind defibrillation should be performed because of the high probability that VF or VT are present. Only about 20% of cardiac arrests are due to "straight-line" asystole, 75% being due to VF. This recommendation (i.e., blind defibrillation) is supported by the well-known fact that the time delay provoked by such measures as applying ECG leads and attempting intubation prior to defibrillation greatly lessens the chance of establishing an effective rhythm. For patients weighing more than 50 kg, the full output of existing defibrillators should be used (usually 400 watt/sec). Patients weighing less than 50 kg should be given 5 watt/sec/kg. Repeated, frequent attempts at defibrillation with 400 watt/sec may cause myocardial damage. Following the restoration of effective rhythm, the patient should be given a bolus of lidocaine and an infusion (2 mg/min) over the next 24 hours as prophylaxis against further ventricular arrhythmias. The decision to infuse bicarbonate must be based on clinical circumstances, particularly the amount of time the patient has spent in VF. Patients with acute MI who are rapidly defibrillated appear to have the same prognosis as those who do not have VF. In fact, patients with VF in the setting of acute MI probably have a better long-term prognosis than those who sustain VF without having suffered an acute MI. (Baum, R. S., Alvarez, H., and Cobb, L. A. Survival after resuscitation from out-of-hospital ventricular fibrillation. *Circulation* 50:1231–1235, 1974.)

Protocol

1. Sinus bradycardia
   - **a. No treatment if the patient is stable.**
   - **b. Heart rates well below 50 beats/min, particularly when associated with chest pain, PVCs, or hypotension, should be treated with intravenous boluses of atropine (0.6–1.0 mg).**
   - **c. If atropine is contraindicated, fails to increase the heart rate, or has to be employed more than three times in 6–12 hours, consider placement of a temporary pacing catheter.**

2. Sinus tachycardia
   - **a. Define underlying etiology: infection, anxiety, pericarditis, hypovolemia, left ventricular failure, pain.**
   - **b. Consider catheterization of the pulmonary artery.**

If PCW is low (<10 mm Hg), infuse volume (e.g., plasma, salt-poor albumin, dextran). If PCW is elevated (>18 mm Hg), intravenous furosemide should be given.

c. If PCW and cardiac output are normal, consider intravenous propranolol (1–3 mg q2–3hr).

3. Atrial fibrillation (AF)
   a. If the ventricular rate is rapid (> 140/min), particularly if there is clinical deterioration (e.g., pulmonary edema, hypotension, chest pain), cardioversion is indicated.
   b. If the ventricular rate is less than 140/min, employ intravenous digoxin (0.25 mg q3–4hr) until the ventricular response is in the range of 70–90/min.
   c. If cardioversion is employed, initiate oral quinidine therapy (200–400 mg q6hr).
4. Atrial flutter
   a. Cardioversion is the preferred treatment for this arrhythmia, since it is frequently difficult to control the ventricular response with digitalis.
5. Paroxysmal atrial tachycardia (PAT)
   a. Sustained PAT should be treated with carotid massage followed by cardioversion should the former maneuver fail. The use of pressor agents, Valsalva maneuvers, and edrophonium is contraindicated.
   b. Following conversion of PAT, and in patients with brief and recurrent episodes of PAT, digoxin and/or quinidine should be given.
6. Premature atrial contractions (PACs)
   a. Other than definition of their etiology (frequently CHF), no therapy is required for PACs.
7. Wandering atrial pacemaker
   a. This arrhythmia is treated in a manner similar to that for PACs.
8. PAT with block
   a. Strongly consider digitalis intoxication.
   b. Monitor serum K+ and administer potassium chloride (KCl) if a low or low-normal serum K+ value is obtained.
   c. Cardioversion should not be attempted if digitalis intoxication is suspected.

9. Junctional rhythms
   a. Slow junctional rhythm is usually a protective escape mechanism and as such need not be treated as long as the ventricular rate is adequate. If the ventricular response is extremely slow or clinical deterioration occurs, consider atropine and/or pacemaker therapy (analogous to sinus bradycardia, above).
   b. Rapid and sustained junctional tachycardia should be treated in a manner similar to that for PAT: carotid massage followed by cardioversion unless digitalis toxicity is suspected.
10. Multifocal atrial tachycardia (MAT)
    a. This arrhythmia is frequently difficult to abort. It is essential to treat the underlying pulmonary and metabolic problems. Cardioversion and digitalis therapy are usually not indicated.
11. AV dissociation
    a. The treatment of this rhythm disturbance depends on its etiology. When the ventricular rate is adequate and the patient is stable, no therapy is necessary.
12. Premature ventricular contractions (PVCs) and ventricular tachycardia (VT)
    a. Give 50–100 mg bolus of lidocaine IV followed by infusion at 2–4 mg/min.
    b. If ventricular ectopy is not significantly suppressed, the infusion rate of lidocaine should be increased to 4 mg/min following an additional bolus of 25–50 mg.
    c. If ventricular ectopy still is not suppressed, add procainamide 50–100 mg IV by slow push q5min until the arrhythmia is abolished, a total of 1.0 g of the drug has been given, or untoward side effects appear (e.g., hypotension or gross widening of the QRS interval). Continue lidocaine infusion while administering procainamide.
    d. If procainamide is effective in abolishing ventricular ectopy, an intravenous infusion should be initiated (1–2 mg/min).
    e. Rarely, ectopy may still not be adequately suppressed. In these instances intravenous propranolol should be considered (0.15 mg/kg—10.5

mg for a 70 kg person—administered by slow IV push at a rate not exceeding 1 mg/min). Hemodynamic monitoring is strongly advised in this setting.

f. **Quinidine may be administered orally (200–400 mg q6h) for chronic suppression of ventricular ectopy. Patients whose ectopy is intermittently persistent or returns following termination of lidocaine therapy may be successfully treated with oral quinidine.**

g. **Dilantin is usually not effective in suppressing ventricular ectopy associated with acute MI. It is a drug of last resort in this setting.**

h. **Sustained ventricular tachycardia should be treated with intravenous lidocaine (as described above), a sharp blow to the precordium, and/or electrical cardioversion, depending upon the clinical state of the patient and the success of previous maneuvers.**

13. **Accelerated idioventricular rhythm (AIVR)**

    a. **Treatment of this arrhythmia is controversial. If the patient is stable no treatment is necessary.**

    b. **If the patient is deteriorating, the rhythm may be overdriven by means of intravenous atropine (0.6–1.0 mg) or suppressed by intravenous lidocaine (50–100 mg IV bolus followed by 2–4 mg/min infusion).**

14. **Ventricular fibrillation (VF)**

    a. **Immediate cardioversion with 400 watt/sec is essential. If reversion to sinus rhythm does not occur, closed-chest cardiac massage, endotracheal intubation and intravenous bicarbonate should be administered, followed by repeated attempts at cardioversion.**

    b. **Following restoration of sinus rhythm, the patient should be treated with intravenous lidocaine for at least 24 hours.**

SUGGESTED READING

Marriot, H. J. L. *Practical Electrocardiography*, 5th ed. Baltimore: Williams & Wilkins Co., 1972.

Constant, J. *Learning Electrocardiography*. Boston: Little, Brown and Co., 1973.

Winkle, R. A., Glantz, S. A., and Harrison, D. C. Pharmacological therapy of ventricular arrhythmias. *Am. J. Cardiol.* 36:629–650, 1975.

Bigger, J. T. Antiarrhythmic drugs in ischemic heart disease. *Hosp. Practice* 69–80, Nov. 1972.

Schamroth, L. How to approach an arrhythmia. *Circulation* 47:420–426, 1973.

12

Pacemakers: Indications for and Technique of Insertion

Currently, there is still uncertainty concerning the short-term and long-term natural history of conduction disturbances in acute MI. Consequently, indications for pacing in this condition are still controversial. Much of the controversy surrounding insertion of temporary prophylactic pacemakers in the setting of acute MI is due to literature that demonstrates that mortality is not clearly affected by this procedure. However, patients who develop serious conduction disturbances in the setting of acute MI can suddenly progress to high grade AV block with very slow ventricular escape rates or even asystole, and it seems reasonable to afford such patients protection from these potentially catastrophic events by the prophylactic placement of a temporary pacemaker. The controversy as to which types of conduction disturbances should be treated with prophylactic pacing exists because the actual probability of the development of life-threatening block is not known. The following criteria reflect a current approach to this as-yet-unresolved problem:

1. Patients with acute MI who develop complete heart block (CHB) with a broad QRS complex and a slow ventricular escape rate are always candidates for a temporary pacemaker.
2. Patients who develop Mobitz Type II conduction disturbance (characterized by a constant P-R interval despite dropped beats) with a wide QRS complex and slow ventricular rate, particularly if associated with an anterior MI and/or fascicular block (left anterior or left posterior hemiblock), are candidates for a temporary pacemaker, even if systemic perfusion is adequate. Such patients usually have permanent destruction of part of the conduction system and are likely to progress to CHB, sometimes suddenly. In patients who de-

velop 2:1 AV block, the site of the conduction disturbance cannot be clearly ascertained by the scalar ECG, and the indication for pacing will depend on the judgment of the physician: the patient with an inferior MI with a narrow QRS, adequate ventricular rate, and no signs or symptoms of hypoperfusion may be observed; whereas pacing is necessary if this patient becomes hypotensive, develops chest pain, or has obvious hypoperfusion. A period of at least three weeks should elapse before deciding to implant a permanent pacemaker in patients with 2:1 or even 3:1 AV block, since complete recovery of normal conduction in such patients may occur when the QRS is narrow.

3. Patients who develop Wenckebach phenomenon are not generally candidates for a pacemaker and need only be observed, provided their blood pressure, mental status, urine output, and other signs of perfusion are adequate. This form of block is usually a temporary event related to ischemia or edema of the AV node which resolves in 24–48 hours, occasionally persisting longer.
4. Patients who develop a new right bundle-branch block (RBBB) with inferior infarction should be observed if they are otherwise stable. Patients who develop a new RBBB with an anterior infarction should be considered for insertion of a temporary pacemaker, since such patients are more likely to proceed to a more advanced form of heart block. Patients who present with an acute MI with a known prior RBBB, or in whom the duration of the conduction disturbance is unknown, should be observed closely, and a pacemaker should be inserted only if further evidence of advanced conduction disturbance arises, e.g., left anterior hemiblock (LAH).
5. Patients with RBBB + LAH or RBBB + LPH (left posterior hemiblock), whether new or previously

documented, who sustain a transmural MI should have a temporary pacemaker placed, since they are sometimes known to progress to CHB without warning.

6. Isolated LAH or LPH, either new or previously documented, does not necessitate insertion of a pacemaker in the setting of acute MI, but such patients should be carefully observed for evidence of further conduction disturbances that may occur and indicate the need for pacing.
7. Patients who develop acute LBBB with an acute MI should have a prophylactic standby pacemaker inserted.
8. Sinus bradycardia unresponsive to repeated doses of atropine and resulting in signs of systemic hypoperfusion (e.g., low urine output, diminished skin temperature, dizziness or mental status changes, hypotension, etc.), chest pain, or serious ventricular arrhythmias (e.g., rapid ventricular tachycardia or ventricular fibrillation) should be treated with a pacemaker. In fact, repeated injections of atropine are not well tolerated by most patients, and a pacemaker should be considered if the bradyarrhythmia requires more than three doses of this drug (see Chapter 11).

Protocol

Indications for Pacing

1. **CHB with slow ventricular rate and wide QRS complex.**
2. **Mobitz type II second degree AV block with associated slow ventricular rate and wide QRS complex.**
    a. **Pacing is particularly important in the setting of anterior infarction or bundle-branch block (RBBB, LBBB).**
    b. **Pacing is usually not indicated for Wenckebach phenomenon (Mobitz type I second-degree AV block).**
3. **New RBBB with anterior infarction.**
4. **RBBB plus LAH or LPH.**
5. **New LBBB.**

6. **Sinus bradycardia or junctional rhythm with slow ventricular rate and clinical signs of hypoperfusion if unresponsive to or requiring repeated doses of atropine.**
7. **Old or age-indeterminate isolated RBBB, LBBB, LAH, or LPH should be observed closely and a pacemaker inserted only if more advanced conduction abnormalities occur.**

Pacemaker catheters may be inserted via the right subclavian, external jugular, or femoral veins by cut-down or Seldinger technique. The position of the lead is probably more stable when these approaches are employed rather than the basilic vein.

Although there are various forms of temporary transvenous pacemakers, including "balloon-tipped" and special lightweight "floating" catheters, the #7 French bipolar USCI pacing catheter* is preferred because it is stable and can be repeatedly sterilized.

Protocol

Insertion of Pacing Catheter via Right Femoral Vein

1. **The patient or next of kin should be informed of the procedure and a note written in the chart explaining the indications and documenting informed consent.**
2. **The patient is placed supine with the right leg apart in a "frog-leg" position. An IV should be secure and running, and the patient should be placed on a special fluoroscopy table. The fluoroscopy image intensifier tube should be turned on, centered over the heart, and tested for adequate imaging before the procedure begins.**
3. **The right groin is prepped with an antiseptic solution and the patient is draped with sterile towels.**
4. **Using sterile technique, the femoral artery is palpated below the inguinal ligament, and the skin area just medial to it is infiltrated intradermally with 1% xylocaine using a 26-gauge needle. A small incision is made with a #11 sharp-pointed scalpel to allow subsequent easy passage of the dilator. A #14 needle**

* Available from U.S. Catheter and Instrument (USCI), P.O. Box 566, Billerica, Massachusetts, 01821

is then used to infiltrate local anesthetic in the region of the femoral vein. Since it is difficult to assess the depth of the vein, small amounts of local anesthetic, about 0.2 ml at a time, should be injected while the needle is advanced slowly.

5. The Seldinger needle, guide wire, connectors, stylets, syringes, etc. should be tested to insure that they are all patent. It is particularly important that the pacemaker pass easily through the thin-walled sheath.
6. When the groin has been anesthetized and the equipment is ready, the operator should advance the Seldinger needle through the previously formed skin incision in a direct line over the femoral vein, just medial to the femoral artery pulsation, at an angle of 45° or less. The needle should be firmly inserted as deeply as it will penetrate.
7. A sterile 10 cc syringe is connected to the Seldinger needle after the stylet has been removed. Suction is then applied to the syringe and the needle and syringe are very slowly withdrawn. A successful puncture is heralded by the appearance of dark venous blood in the syringe.
8. At this point the syringe is disconnected and the soft tip of the guide wire is inserted through the lumen of the needle provided there is still free flow of blood from the needle. The guide wire should pass easily through the Seldinger needle and into the femoral vein. If it does not, the wire should *not* be forced since the tip of the needle may be extraluminal.
9. Once the wire is securely in the vein, the needle is removed and the wire remains. A firm dilator is then passed over the wire, making sure that the firm tip of the guide wire is held beyond the blunt end of the dilator.
10. The dilator is then firmly introduced into the vein over the wire, preparing a pathway for the insertion of the sheath and pacing catheter.
11. When the dilator has been passed several times through the skin and into the vein, the thin-walled sheath is inserted with the dilator in a firm rotating fashion. The dilator and wire are then removed, and dark venous blood should flow easily from the sheath.
12. The pacing catheter is then inserted through the

sheath into the femoral vein and inferior vena cava (IVC) where it is visualized by fluoroscopy. The sheath may then be removed from the vein, and the catheter advanced to the right atrium.

13. Under fluoroscopic control, a loop is formed in the right atrium, and the catheter is manipulated across the tricuspid valve and into the apex of the right ventricle.
14. The catheter is then connected to the external pacing generator. The pacemaker is then turned on and the *threshold* or the least amount of milliamps necessary to consistently capture the ventricle is determined. The groin is then dressed and the catheter secured with adhesive tape to the right leg.
15. Ideally, the initial threshold should allow consistent capture at a milliamperage (MA) energy setting of less than 1 MA. The amperage should then be set at about twice the threshold. If more than 5–6 milliamps are required for consistent capture, further positioning of the lead should be attempted. Such high milliamperage may be dangerous and is more likely to cause VF in an ischemic myocardium. The pacemaker should be set on the demand mode at a rate sufficient to overdrive ectopic foci, usually about 70–80 beats/min.
16. Immediately after catheter insertion, a complete 12-lead ECG should be recorded and a chest x-ray should be obtained. The threshold required to pace should be checked daily by the physician by turning the MA down to the point of noncapture. This threshold value is recorded in the patient's chart. The MA is kept at twice this level. It is not uncommon for the threshold to increase slightly over the first 24 to 48 hours after the pacemaker is inserted.
17. Long-term permanent pacing should be considered in selective cases, since there is data to indicate that patients who survive a serious conduction disturbance during an acute MI (e.g., LBBB, LAH, and RBBB) with persistence of that disturbance into the recovery phase, may have a high incidence of sudden death if implantation of a permanent pacemaker is not performed.

SUGGESTED READING

Resnekov, L., and Lipp, H. Pacemaking and acute myocardial infarction. *Prog. Cardiovasc. Dis.* 14:475–494, 1972.

Nimetz, A. A., Shubrooks, S. J., Jr., Hutter, A. M., and DeSanctis, R. W. The significance of bundle branch block during acute myocardial infarction. *Am. Heart J.* 90:439–444, 1975.

Waugh, R. A., Wagner, G. S., Haney, T. L., Rosati, R. A., and Morris, J. J. Immediate and remote prognostic significance of fascicular block during acute myocardial infarction. *Circulation* 47:765–777, 1973.

Meltzer, L. E., and Kitchell, J. R., eds. *Current Concepts of Cardiac Pacing and Cardioversion.* Philadelphia: The Charles Press, 1971.

Treatment of Left Ventricular Failure Complicating Myocardial Infarction

Elevation of left ventricular end-diastolic pressure (LVEDP) is very common in acute MI. However, elevated LVEDP does not always result in clinical left ventricular failure, i.e., rales and left ventricular S_3 gallop. There are two presumptive causes for the LVEDP elevation in acute MI: (1) left ventricular failure with compensatory increase in left ventricular end-diastolic volume (Starling's Law), or (2) decreased left ventricular compliance (increased stiffness of the left ventricular wall) with normal left ventricular end-diastolic volume. Frequently, elevated LVEDP is the result of a combination of these two factors. The practical consequences of these two etiologies for elevation of LVEDP are: patients with rales in whom elevation of LVEDP is judged to be the result of decreased compliance (i.e., normal heart size, absence of S_3 gallop, normal cardiac output) should be treated with diuretics, whereas patients whose elevated LVEDP results from elevated end-diastolic volume (i.e., enlarged heart, S_3 gallop, decreased cardiac output) should receive digitalis and diuretics. Further assistance in differentiating these two forms of *left ventricular failure* can be obtained by means of chest roentgenography (for heart size) and echocardiography (for left ventricular end-diastolic internal dimension).

The clinical definition of left ventricular failure following acute MI is as follows: moist rales at the lung bases which persist after a vigorous cough often accompanied by tachycardia, an S_3, tachypnea, and dyspnea. Chest roentgenography usually demonstrates vascular blurring, dilatation, or parenchymal clouding in such patients.

Protocol

1. **If the heart is of normal size on the chest x-ray, the initial therapeutic intervention should be small intra-**

venous doses (20 mg) of furosemide. If the heart is enlarged on the chest x-ray, the patient should be given digoxin 0.25 mg t.i.d. for 2 days followed by maintenance digoxin at 0.25 mg/day (maintenance dosage depends on adequacy of renal function). Additional intravenous furosemide is given as required.

a. Patients who have an adequate diuresis from furosemide but continue to manifest signs of left ventricular failure should be digitalized regardless of heart size on the chest x-ray.
b. If tachycardia develops after adequate furosemide diuresis either before or after digoxin therapy, a pulmonary-artery balloon catheter should be inserted to measure left ventricular filling pressure (see Chapters 11 and 24).
   (1) If the tachycardia is secondary to overvigorous diuresis (PCW less than 12 mm Hg), colloid (albumin, plasma, or low molecular weight dextran) should be infused until the wedge pressure is approximately 18 mm Hg.
   (2) If the tachycardia has occurred in the face of adequate left ventricular filling pressures (PCW of 12 mm Hg or greater), the digitalis therapy described above (if not already done) should be initiated.
   (3) If the tachycardia has occurred in the face of PCWs greater than 20 mm Hg, digitalis therapy should be continued or initiated and supplemental intravenous doses of furosemide employed until the wedge pressure falls to approximately 18 mm Hg.
   (4) If tachycardia and/or signs of left ventricular failure persist despite digitalis and repeated furosemide therapy (or PCW remains >20 mm Hg), nitroprusside or nitroglycerin paste therapy is initiated.
      (a) Nitroprusside infusion (systemic arterial and pulmonary arterial pressure monitoring mandatory) is begun at 15 μg/min and increased at 3–5 min intervals until the PCW falls below 18 mm Hg. Systolic arterial pressure should not fall below 95–100 mm Hg. It is rarely neces-

sary to infuse more than 200 μg/min of nitroprusside. Nitroglycerin paste is applied at 4–6 hr intervals starting with ½–1 inch and gradually increasing the dose (more than 2 inches q4h is rarely needed) until the wedge pressure falls below 18 mm Hg.

(b) Patients who do not manifest tachycardia or severe left ventricular failure, but who nevertheless have persistent modest findings of left ventricular failure, may be treated with nitroglycerin paste without pulmonary arterial pressure monitoring. In addition, patients who are treated with nitroprusside for left ventricular failure can frequently be weaned from the nitroprusside infusion with gradually increasing doses of nitroglycerin paste or oral vasodilators. Start the nitroglycerin paste at ½ inch q4–6h and increase daily to a maximum of 2 inches q4h. Systolic blood pressure should not fall below 95–100 mm Hg.

2. Occasional patients with severe, persistent left ventricular failure (usually frank or borderline pulmonary edema) can be stabilized with intra-aortic balloon or external counterpulsation. Such patients almost invariably require cardiac surgical intervention (e.g., coronary artery bypass graft, infarctectomy) during the same hospitalization.

SUGGESTED READING

Rackley, C. E., and Russell, R. D. Left ventricular function in acute myocardial infarction and its clinical significance. *Circulation* 45:231–244, 1972.

Crexells, C., Chatterjee, K., Forrester, J. S., Dikshit, K., and Swan, H. J. C. Optimal level of filling pressure in the left side of the heart in acute myocardial infarction. *N. Engl. J. Med.* 289:1263–1266, 1973.

Franciosa, J. A., Guiha, N. H., Limas, C. J., Paz, S., and Cohn, J. N. Arterial pressure as a determinant of left ventricular filling pressure after acute myocardial infarction. *Am. J. Cardiol.* 34:506–512, 1974.

Chatterjee, K., and Swan, H. J. C. Vasodilator therapy in acute myocardial infarction. *Mod. Concepts Cardiovasc. Dis.* 43:119–124, 1974.

Armstrong, P. W., Walker, D. C., Burton, J. R., and Parker, J. O. Vasodilator therapy in acute myocardial infarction: a comparison of sodium nitroprusside and nitroglycerin. *Circulation* 52:1118–1122, 1975.

Mantle, J. A., Russell, R. O., Jr., Moraski, R. E., and Rackley, C. E. Isosorbide dinitrate for the relief of severe heart failure after myocardial infarction. *Am. J. Cardiol.* 37:263–268, 1976.

Rahimtoola, S. H. Digitalis in acute myocardial infarction: help or hazard? *Ann. Intern. Med.* 82:234–240, 1975.

Wolk, M. J., Scheidt, S., and Killip, T. Heart failure complicating acute myocardial infarction. *Circulation* 45:1125–1138, 1972.

14

Treatment of Acute Mitral Regurgitation and Ventricular Septal Rupture

A loud systolic murmur associated with signs and symptoms of severe left ventricular failure developing in a patient with an acute MI is highly suggestive of acute mitral regurgitation or rupture of the ventricular septum.

Patients who rupture an entire papillary muscle deteriorate rapidly despite intensive medical management. Papillary muscle dysfunction or the rupture of only one or two chordae tendineae can be associated with severe left ventricular failure, but the patient's demise is not quite as precipitous as with rupture of an entire papillary muscle. Patients with rupture (tear) of the ventricular septum have a clinical course similar to that seen with papillary muscle dysfunction or subtotal papillary muscle rupture.

It is frequently difficult to differentiate between the murmurs of acute mitral regurgitation and ventricular septal rupture. A pulmonary arterial catheter should be inserted in all patients suspected of having sustained one of these two complications. An arterial line is almost always required as well. A Foley catheter is frequently helpful in monitoring urine output in these critically ill patients.

Protocol

1. **Pulmonary arterial and systemic arterial catheters are inserted. Serial, duplicate 2-cc blood samples should be obtained in heparinized syringes from the superior vena cava, right atrium, right ventricle, and pulmonary artery as the balloon catheter is advanced. These samples should be free of air bubbles, capped and preserved on ice until percent oxygen saturation determinations can be performed. It is not necessary to discontinue supplemental inspiratory oxygen.**
2. **The presence of a significant increase (or "step-up") in**

right ventricular oxygen saturation (as compared with right atrial values) is diagnostic of ventricular septal rupture (see 3 below). The absence of a step-up combined with the presence of large V waves in the PCW tracing implies significant acute mitral regurgitation.

3. In order to determine if a patient has a significant oxygen step-up, blood samples are obtained from the superior vena cava, right atrium, right ventricle, and pulmonary artery as described under item 1. All samples have their oxygen content calculated as follows:

$$\text{Oxygen content of the sample in volumes \%} = \text{hemoglobin (g\%)} \times 1.39 \times \text{\% saturation of the sample}$$

A difference of greater than 1 volume percent between the right atrium and the right ventricle signifies a significant left-to-right shunt from a ventricular septal rupture. The amount of blood shunting left to right can be calculated from the following formulas:

a. Left-to-right shunt = pulmonary blood flow − systemic blood flow.

b. Pulmonary blood flow

$$= \frac{\text{oxygen consumption}}{\text{(arterial blood } O_2 \text{ content)} - \text{(pulmonary arterial blood } O_2 \text{ content)}}$$

c. Systemic blood flow

$$= \frac{\text{oxygen consumption}}{\text{(arterial blood } O_2 \text{ content)} - \text{(right atrial arterial blood } O_2 \text{ content)}}$$

Oxygen consumption is determined with a Douglas bag and the help of the Catheterization Laboratory or may be assumed to be 125 cc/min/M^2. The patient's body surface area in M^2 can be easily determined from a nomogram if one knows the individual's height and weight (see Appendix 3).

4. The treatment of acute mitral regurgitation (MR) and ventricular septal rupture (VSD) is similar. It consists of attempts to "compensate" the left ventricle and allow for elective surgical correction at a later date (usually three months).
   a. Milder forms of MR and VSD produce left ventricu-

lar failure that can be successfully controlled with digitalis and diuretic therapy.

b. More severe forms of MR and VSD are associated with considerable degrees of left ventricular failure (PCWs of >20 mm Hg), requiring more aggressive management.

   (1) A nitroprusside infusion should be initiated (intra-arterial pressure monitoring essential) at 15 μg/min and the drip rate increased at intervals of 3–5 min until the PCW falls below 18 mm Hg. Systolic arterial pressure should not fall below 95–100 mm Hg. It is rarely necessary to infuse more than 200 μg/min of nitroprusside.
   (2) If the patient is hypotensive, most authorities feel that nitroprusside is contraindicated and dopamine infusion should be instituted as described in the protocol for cardiogenic shock (see Chapter 15). Some authorities have employed a combination of dopamine and nitroprusside in these patients. This form of therapy is still under investigation.
   (3) Intra-aortic balloon or external counterpulsation is strongly recommended unless contraindicated (e.g., severe obliterative peripheral vascular disease). The counterpulsation team is mobilized by consultation with the Cardiology Service. The director of the CCU should be informed of the presence of the patient in the Unit.
   (4) Cardiac surgical repair (mitral valve replacement or VSD closure) are ideally postponed until the patient is over the acute phase of the MI. However, some patients who would not otherwise have survived can be salvaged by emergency catheterization and surgery. Coronary artery bypass grafts are usually performed along with the repair procedure (see Chapter 25).

SUGGESTED READING

Mundth, E. D., Buckley, J. J., Daggett, W. M., Sanders, C. A., and Austen, W. G. Surgery for complications of acute myocardial infarction. *Circulation* 45:1279–1291, 1972.

Giuliani, E. R., Danielson, G. K., Pluth, J. R., Odyniec, N. A., and Wallace, R. B. Postinfarction ventricular septal rupture: surgical considerations and results. *Circulation* 49:455–459, 1974.

Braunwald, E. Mitral regurgitation: physiologic, clinical and surgical considerations. *N. Engl. J. Med.* 281:425–433, 1969.

Burch, G. E., DePasquale, N. P., and Phillips, J. H. The syndrome of papillary muscle dysfunction. *Am. Heart J.* 75:399–415, 1968.

15

Treatment of Suspected Cardiogenic Shock

Cardiogenic shock (CGS) is the most dreaded complication of acute MI with a mortality frequently in excess of 90%. This entity occurs when approximately 40% of the left ventricular myocardium is rendered nonfunctional by necrosis and ischemia. The clinical criteria defining CGS are clearly important if accurate assessment of various forms of therapy is to be achieved. The incidence of CGS and the results of therapy vary in different clinical centers because of differences in the definition of CGS. The criteria stated below for CGS reflect current established definitions of this entity.

1. Patients are diagnosed as having cardiogenic shock (CGS) by the following criteria:
   a. The diagnosis of MI by the usual clinical data (i.e., history, physical examination, ECG).
   b. Systolic blood pressure less than 90 mm Hg by cuff on two successive determinations. However, a higher pressure (e.g., 100 mm Hg) may occur in patients previously hypertensive.
   c. Urine output less than 20–30 cc/hr.
   d. Absence of other causes of hypotension such as:
      (1) Overenthusiastic dosage of quinidine, procainamide, and/or antihypertensive medications
      (2) Arrhythmias
      (3) Significant disorders of electrolytes, acid-base, and arterial blood gases
      (4) Dehydration or bradycardia-hypotension syndrome (see below)
   e. Presence of clinical signs of shock such as depressed mentation and peripheral vasoconstriction (e.g., pallid or mottled, cool, clammy skin).

Protocol

1. All patients with suspected CGS should have a pulmonary arterial catheter placed via the neck, arm, or leg (see Chapter 24). PCW (confirmed by a similar pulmonary arterial diastolic pressure unless the patient has significant COPD) should be 15–18 mm Hg or more. Patients with values less than this are either dehydrated (e.g., from chronic diuretic use) or have the bradycardia-hypotension syndrome (Bezold-Jarisch reflex—particularly common with inferior MIs). The latter two groups of patients should be infused with either albumin, plasma, or low-molecular-weight dextran until a wedge pressure of approximately 18 mm Hg is obtained. Dextrose in water and saline are NOT recommended for volume therapy since these latter agents usually leak across capillary membranes and hence are only transient in their effectiveness. Significant bradycardia should be treated with IV atropine or pacing (see Chapters 11 and 12).
2. All patients with suspected CGS should have an arterial line placed with the lumen as close to the aorta as possible. Peripheral arterial pressures (e.g., radial artery) can be misleading. Relatively long catheters inserted from the brachial or femoral arteries are preferred. Slow, continuous, low-dose heparin infusion (1 unit/cc in 5% D/W or saline) should be instituted through both arterial and pulmonary arterial catheters. A Foley catheter should also be inserted to aid in monitoring urine output.
3. While systemic arterial and pulmonary arterial lines are being introduced into the patient in order to assess the severity of the shock state and the left ventricular filling pressure, it is frequently prudent to support the systemic blood pressure pharmacologically with dopamine or norepinephrine (see item 4a below). If the patient is subsequently found (by pulmonary arterial catheterization) to be hypovolemic, these pressor agents can be gradually tapered while appropriate volume therapy is administered.
4. Treatment of patients in whom intra-arterial pressures and clinical data support the diagnosis of CGS:
   a. A trial of dopamine infusion is instituted, starting with 2–5 μg/kg/min and increasing the dose to 20–50 μg/kg/min if inadequate response is ob-

tained. If an inadequate response is obtained with dopamine, a trial infusion of norepinephrine (Levophed) is warranted, dosage 2–8 μg/min (N.B.: total dosage is 2–8 μg/min—NOT 2–8 μg/kg/min). Isoproterenol is contraindicated (see Chapter 20).

b. Mobilization of the intra-aortic balloon (or external) counterpulsation team should be considered. Cardiology should be consulted (if not already done) and they will notify the director of the CCU of the presence of a patient in CGS in the unit.

5. Patients in CGS are felt by certain authorities to benefit from digitalis, diuretics, and/or anticoagulants. The use of digitalis, diuretics, and anticoagulants in such patients is controversial.

6. Patients with CGS frequently benefit from intra-aortic balloon or external counterpulsation. Some patients in CGS are candidates for emergency coronary artery bypass grafts (CABG). The decision to catheterize such patients with an eye to performing an emergency CABG procedure must be individualized. Patients in whom the CGS state is severe, or who fail to improve rapidly over the initial 24–48 hours after initiation of counterpulsation, should be considered for CABG. Patients with mechanical complications of acute MI (i.e., MR or VSD) associated with CGS frequently benefit from surgical intervention.

   a. Patients should be transferred to the Catheterization Laboratory and the procedure should be performed during counterpulsation. The patient may return to the CCU following the catheterization or he/she may proceed directly to the operating room (see Chapter 25).

SUGGESTED READING

Page, D. L., Caulfield, J. J., Kastor, J. A., DeSanctis, R. W., and Saunders, C. A. Myocardial changes associated with cardiogenic shock. *N. Engl. J. Med.* 285:133–137, 1971.

Alonso, D. R., Scheidt, S., Post, M., and Killip, T. Pathophysiology of cardiogenic shock: quantification of myocardial necrosis, clinical, pathologic and electrocardiographic correlations. *Circulation* 48:588–596, 1973.

Kuhn, L. A. Shock in myocardial infarction—medical treatment. *Am. J. Cardiol.* 26:578–587, 1970.
Gunnar, R. M., Loeb, H. S. Use of drugs in cardiogenic shock due to acute myocardial infarction. *Circulation* 45:1111–1124, 1972.

16

Treatment of Hypertension Complicating Acute Myocardial Infarction

Arterial blood pressure as it relates to systolic left ventricular wall tension is an important determinant of myocardial oxygen consumption. Therefore, hypertension in the setting of acute MI may be detrimental. Moreover, increased left ventricular systolic pressure predisposes patients with acute MI to rupture of the left ventricular free wall.

It is not uncommon for patients to be hypertensive early in the course of acute MI, particularly in the setting of anterior MI. This pressor response may be mediated via a sympathetic nervous reflex.

Protocol

1. **Patients with acute MI, diagnosed by the usual clinical data (i.e., history, physical examination, ECG) who are hypertensive (BP > 145/95 mm Hg by cuff) on admission to the CCU should be treated as follows:**
   a. **Patients with chest pain should be given sufficient sedation (diazepam) and intravenous morphine sulfate or demerol to abolish the pain. Analgesics should be given repeatedly q 15-20 min in moderate doses (e.g., morphine 5 mg) until pain is relieved. Pentazocine should be avoided because it can elevate blood pressure.**
   b. **Patients with signs and symptoms of left ventricular failure should be treated with intravenous furosemide: starting dose 20 mg IV (see Chapter 13).**
      (1) **Patients in pulmonary edema should be treated with the usual measures: morphine, furosemide, tourniquets, etc.**
2. **Patients who remain hypertensive (BP > 145/95 mm Hg by cuff) 30–60 min after chest pain and left ventricular failure have been relieved should be treated as follows:**
   a. **Administration of intravenous furosemide (20–40 mg) if not already done.**
   b. **Administration of isosorbide dinitrate, 5 mg sublingual (SL) or chewable; recheck blood pressure in**

5 minutes. If an adequate hypotensive response is obtained, the patient is placed on SL or oral isosorbide dinitrate at sufficient intervals to control the blood pressure (e.g., 5 mg q2 or 4h). Blood pressure is monitored by cuff at frequent intervals in order to decide the frequency of dosage. Vascular headaches associated with isosorbide therapy can usually be suppressed with acetaminophen or aspirin.

c. If the first dose of isosorbide dinitrate fails to adequately lower the blood pressure in 5 minutes, a second dose should be given.

3. If two doses of isosorbide dinitrate and a significant diuresis fail to lower the blood pressure to satisfactory levels and proper sedation and alleviation of pain have been accomplished, some authorities advocate more aggressive antihypertensive therapy: intra-arterial blood pressure monitoring and administration of intravenous nitroprusside.
   a. Nitroprusside infusions are initiated at 15 μg/min and the drip rate increased at intervals of 3–5 min until the arterial pressure drops to normal levels (systolic blood pressure 100–120 mm Hg). It is rarely necessary to infuse more than 200 μg/min of nitroprusside.
   b. Patients who require nitroprusside therapy should be started concomitantly on oral antihypertensive drugs such as methyldopa and a diuretic. In patients without evidence of left ventricular failure, propranolol is an excellent adjunct to the antihypertensive regimen. Clonidine may be contraindicated in the immediate postinfarction period (particularly following nitroprusside infusions) since significant hypotensive episodes can occur with the combination of these two medicines in the setting of acute MI. Oral antihypertensives should always be started with low doses and increased daily by small amounts. Nitroprusside infusion can be tapered as the blood pressure comes under control. Important side effects may occur as a result of nitroprusside therapy. Significant thiocyanate levels can be generated during prolonged nitroprusside therapy, resulting in toxic symptoms (e.g., fatigue, anorexia, disorientation, psychosis, muscle spasms). If toxic symptoms

occur or thiocyanate levels exceed 10 mg%, the drug should be discontinued.

c. **Intravenous nitroprusside therapy for hypertension in the setting of acute MI is controversial. Its net effect on experimental and clinical infarct size may be variable. Definition of the exact role of nitroprusside in this setting must await further clinical data.**

d. **Many authorities advocate a traditional oral antihypertensive regimen for patients with acute MI who remain hypertensive despite adequate sedation, diuresis, analgesia, and nitrate therapy.**

SUGGESTED READING

Palmer, R. F., and Lasseter, K. C. Drug therapy—sodium nitroprusside. *N. Engl. J. Med.* 292:294–297, 1975.

Shell, W. E., Sobel, B. E. Protection of jeopardized ischemic myocardium by reduction of ventricular afterload. *N. Engl. J. Med.* 291:482–486, 1974.

Watanabe, T., Covell, J. W., Maroko, P. R., Braunwald, E., and Ross, J., Jr. Effects of increased arterial pressure and positive inotropic agents on the severity of myocardial ischemia in the acutely depressed heart. *Am. J. Cardiol.* 30:371–377, 1972.

17

Treatment of Unstable Angina and Coronary Insufficiency

Cardiologists do not agree as to the appropriate criteria or even the best name for unstable angina and coronary insufficiency (also called crescendo angina, preinfarction angina, or intermediate syndrome). The following criteria reflect current definitions:

1. Patients with unstable angina have recurring anginal-chest pain at rest with episodes lasting 20–30 min or more. At least two episodes occurring within seven days of the current hospitalization (or during it) are required in order to make the diagnosis. The pain is usually more severe than exertional angina. The anginal episode may respond to nitrates (usually more than a single dose) but frequently requires opiates for relief. There are no precipitating factors (e.g., heavy meals, emotion, etc.). Patients with simply a change in the pattern of previously stable angina, angina of recent onset, or angina decubitus are not included in this category unless they meet the other criteria stated above. Likewise, subjects with a single episode of pain are not included. In the past, patients with unstable angina were frequently labeled as having "severe coronary insufficiency."
2. At least one episode of pain should be associated with characteristic ischemic ST-T changes on the electrocardiogram. Many patients will have fluctuating ECG changes; others will develop persistent changes.
3. Nondiagnostic serum enzyme changes, i.e., normal CPK, SGOT, and LDH.

Protocol

1. **Patients who meet the diagnostic criteria stated above must be admitted to the hospital and placed on bed/**

chair activity with bathroom or commode privileges. It is highly desirable that such patients be monitored.

2. Diet should be light (e.g., 1,500 calorie, low cholesterol) and Valsalva maneuvers at stool should be discouraged (stool softeners are recommended) (see Chapter 6).
3. The initiation of digitalis therapy is usually contraindicated in these patients unless they have clearcut clinical/radiologic evidence of left ventricular failure or cardiomegaly. Previously instituted digitalis therapy should be continued or discontinued, depending upon the above-mentioned indications.
4. It is vital that a reassuring, quiet, and stable environment be created for the patient. This requires appropriate physician and nurse demeanor and restriction of visitors, telephone calls, etc. A mild sedative is frequently helpful (e.g., diazepam, chlordiazepoxide, etc.). Supplemental inspiratory oxygen may also be desirable.
5. Some authorities advocate a trial of diuretic therapy, particularly if the patient has decubitus or nocturnal angina as one of the manifestations of unstable angina.
6. The mainstay of therapy for such patients is beta blockade and nitrates. Propranolol should be started in low doses (e.g., 10 mg q.i.d.) providing no contraindications exist: LV failure, asthma, COPD with bronchospasm, conduction defects by ECG. The propranolol dose should be gradually increased each day until a dose of 80–360 mg/day is achieved. Propranolol therapy is monitored by observing the heart-rate response. Adequately treated patients usually have heart rates of 40–60 beats/min at rest.

   Nitrate therapy may be started concomitantly with propranolol. A good starting dose is 5 mg of isosorbide dinitrate chewed or SL q.i.d. Nitroglycerin paste is also quite satisfactory and has a longer duration of action than sublingual nitroglycerin. The initial dose here is ½ in. q4–6h. Nitroglycerin paste can be increased to 2 in. q4h while the patient is awake, as tolerated. The paste should be spread over a 6 × 6-in. area. Systolic blood pressure should not be allowed to fall below 90–100 mm Hg on combined propranolol and nitrate therapy. Frequently patients will tolerate

marked sinus bradycardia (e.g., 40 beats/min) surprisingly well.

7. **Most patients rapidly become pain-free on the regimen outlined above. Once rest angina has been abolished, the patient is gradually permitted to walk. If he/she tolerates ambulation, he/she may be discharged to prompt outpatient follow-up on the same regimen that was used in the hospital. It is important to instruct the patient to RETURN to the hospital if he/she suffers attacks of rest angina or frequent anginal attacks resulting from minimal exertion.**
8. **Patients whose anginal attacks at rest or with minimal exertion continue are candidates for catheterization followed by coronary artery bypass surgery (CABG).**
9. **If the patient continues to manifest considerable amounts of angina despite hospitalization and adequate medical therapy, intra-aortic balloon or external counterpulsation can be initiated to stabilize the patient prior to cardiac catheterization and immediate CABG surgery (see Chapter 25).**

SUGGESTED READING

Krauss, K. R., Hutter, A. M., and DeSanctis, R. W. Acute coronary insufficiency—course and follow-up. *Circulation* (Suppl.) 40, 41:I-66–I-71, 1972.

Harrison, D. C., and Shumway, N. Evaluation and surgery for impending myocardial infarction. *Hosp. Practice* 49–58, Dec, 1972.

Cannom, D. S., Harrison, D. C., and Schroeder, J. S. Hemodynamic observations in patients with unstable angina pectoris. *Am. J. Cardiol.* 33:17–22, 1974.

Fischl, S. J., Herman, M. V., and Gorlin, R. The intermediate coronary syndrome—clinical, angiographic, and therapeutic aspects. *N. Engl. J. Med.* 288:1193–1198, 1973.

Fowler, N. O. "Preinfarctional" angina—a need for an objective definition and for a controlled clinical trial of its management. *Circulation* 44:755–758, 1971.

Favaloro, R. G., Effler, D. B., Cheanvechai, C., Quint, R. A., and Sones, F. M., Jr. Acute coronary insufficiency (impending myocardial infarction and myocardial infarction)—surgical treatment by the saphenous vein graft technique. *Am. J. Cardiol.* 28:598–607, 1971.

18

Treatment of Angina in the Immediate Postinfarction Period

Patients with angina in the immediate (first three weeks) postinfarction period should be treated in a manner similar to that employed for patients with unstable angina (see Chapter 17). It is not unusual for patients with acute MI to have some residual chest discomfort for 2–3 days after the acute event. Moreover, a significant number of patients with myocardial infarction develop early (first 72 hours) or late (seven days to several months) pericarditis (see Chapter 19). Pain from the latter condition can easily be confused with angina pectoris unless the characteristic positional (pain worse on recumbency and improved on sitting) and pleuritic (pain worse on inspiration) qualities of pericarditic discomfort are elicited. Pericardial rubs are usually evanescent; hence the absence of a rub does not rule out the diagnosis of pericarditis.

Protocol

1. If a patient develops chest discomfort suggestive of myocardial ischemia (particularly if associated with exertion such as the morning toilet); and if such pain occurs between 2 and 21 days post infarction; and if pericarditis seems unlikely, then it should be assumed that the patient is suffering from angina pectoris immediately post infarction.

2. Signs and symptoms of left ventricular failure should be sought, since a dilated left ventricle with a high filling pressure has a higher myocardial oxygen consumption than the same ventricle at a smaller volume and with a lower filling pressure.

   a. Patients who are felt to have significant left ventricular failure (e.g., rales, S_3, cardiomegaly and/or pulmonary vascular redistribution by x-ray, elevated filling pressures) should be treated with digitalis and diuretic preparations as described in Chapter 13.

b. If angina still occurs in the absence of, or following adequate treatment for, left ventricular failure, then propranolol and nitrate therapy should be initiated as described in Chapter 17. All anginal episodes should be promptly treated with sublingual nitroglycerin (with 2–3 repeated doses if necessary and if the blood pressure is adequate). Activity should be moderately reduced until adequate propranolol and nitrate dosage has been achieved (propranolol 20–40 mg PO q6h; isosorbide dinitrate 5–10 mg chewed or SL q2–3h). Thereafter, activity may be increased again to see if the episodes of angina pectoris recur.

c. If angina pectoris recurs with minimal or very modest activity it is probable that anginal attacks will occur even more frequently at home following discharge from the hospital. Therefore, such patients should be considered for cardiac catheterization and coronary artery bypass surgery (see Chapter 25).

d. Coronary artery surgery is best performed at least three months following an acute MI. If the patient with angina pectoris can decrease his activity sufficiently so that anginal episodes are few, of modest intensity, and rapidly relieved by nitroglycerin, then surgery can safely be delayed until 12 weeks post infarction. Clearly, many patients will have angina of such a refractory nature that surgery cannot be delayed. The timing of catheterization and surgery in such patients must be individualized.

SUGGESTED READING

See references following Chapter 17.

19

Treatment of Miscellaneous Complications of Acute Myocardial Infarction: Pericarditis, Pulmonary Embolism, Arterial Embolism, and Myocardial Rupture

PERICARDITIS

The incidence of clinical pericarditis occurring in the setting of acute MI varies from 7 to 42%. It generally implies a transmural infarction and may be seen with posterior-inferior infarctions as well as anterior infarctions. The key physical finding is a pericardial friction rub, which may be audible a few hours after the onset of pain, but is most commonly heard on the second or third day. The rub may appear intermittently, persisting briefly at each appearance. It is wise to have its presence confirmed by another observer because of its capricious nature. The pericardial friction rub's three components are related to atrial contraction, ventricular systole, and rapid ventricular filling. Not all components are necessarily present, however, and the only audible sign can be a soft, scratchy systolic sound. The rub is usually best heard just inside the apical impulse, or along the left sternal border. There is usually associated pleuritic chest pain that is relieved by sitting up. There may be a low-grade fever (up to 102°) and sinus tachycardia. Usually the discomfort of pericarditis is of brief duration.

The pain may be confused with extension of the infarction, pulmonary embolism, or bronchopneumonia. Treatment can be important when the patient is uncomfortable because it lowers the heart rate and alleviates pain and anxiety. Rarely, patients go on to develop chronic recurrent pericarditis associated with pneumonitis (Dressler's syndrome). This may last from months to years, is thought to be autoimmune in nature, and is usually treated in a manner similar to acute pericarditis.

Protocol

1. **Indomethacin (100–200 mg/day) or salicylates (650 mg q.i.d.) should be used along with low-sodium antacids.**
2. **Prolonged corticosteroid therapy is to be avoided in pericarditis associated with acute MI since there is evidence to suggest that it may result in aneurysm formation and even myocardial rupture due to delayed healing of the infarction. Prolonged severe Dressler's syndrome refractory to salicylate and indomethacin therapy can be treated with moderate doses of corticosteroids (prednisone 60 mg PO q.d. for 2–3 weeks). Withdrawal of steroids should be very gradual (over a 6–8-week period) in patients with Dressler's syndrome, since pericarditis commonly recurs.**
3. **Anticoagulants should be avoided, particularly when the rub is loud and diffuse and persists longer than a few days. Although the risk of hemopericardium is small, a less than therapeutic range of anticoagulation is recommended if such agents must be used.**

PULMONARY EMBOLISM (P.E.)

This occurs in an uncertain number of patients with acute MI, but the incidence is relatively small. It is important to recognize it, however, because it may provoke hemodynamic embarrassment or atrial arrhythmias. Recognition of this great masquerader is difficult and requires a high index of suspicion. It is a particularly difficult diagnosis to make in the setting of acute MI where chest pain, hypoxia, and dyspnea are already present. Recurrent episodes of weakness, sweating, dyspnea, and arrhythmias in the absence of hypertension should alert one to the diagnosis. Episodic weakness, sweating, dyspnea, and arrhythmias associated with hypertension or hypotension can be due to pheochromocytoma. If the patient's condition permits, a lung scan should be performed. This may prove extremely useful, because a negative lung scan excludes a significant pulmonary embolus. A positive scan supports the diagnosis but is not sensitive enough by itself to make it definite. Such patients can undergo pulmonary angiography although this is done at an increased risk. Angiography should only be performed in this setting if a significant alteration in therapy depends on the results of this test.

The electrocardiogram may show a right axis shift, acute RBBB, or right atrial enlargement. These changes usually require massive pulmonary embolism, are nonspecific, and are frequently seen in acute MI without P.E. They are therefore not very helpful. If the clinical index of suspicion is high, and if the lung scan is clearly positive, the patient should be treated with anticoagulants. Various guidelines for therapeutic heparin therapy can be employed and there are numerous recommendations on how to give the drug.

Protocol

1. **If continuous intravenous heparin administration is decided upon, a loading dose of 5,000–10,000 units is given intravenously, followed by an infusion usually averaging 25,000–30,000 units per 24 hours, the dose being adjusted on the basis of an activated partial thromboplastin time determined at least once daily (a value of 50–80 sec is therapeutic).**
2. **For the intermittent intravenous method of heparin therapy an average dose of 5,000 units every 4 hr will usually suffice, although the dose may vary from 2,500 units to 10,000 units (150 units/kg/24hr). Heparin therapy should be given for 7–10 days, the time required for the thrombus to become adherent to the vein wall, and oral anticoagulants should then be started. The administration of heparin and oral warfarin derivatives should overlap for 3–5 days in order to allow the antithrombic effect of the oral agent to occur. Warfarin should be given for at least three months.**

ARTERIAL EMBOLISM

Mural thrombi may form at the site of endocardial injury and be discharged into the circulation as emboli. This infrequent complication may result in stroke, infarction of various organs, or symptoms of acute arterial insufficiency in an extremity. Embolism to the central nervous system may present with fleeting neurological signs or dense hemiparesis, usually sudden in onset. The Neurology Service should be consulted, and the decision concerning anticoagulation should be based on the presence of or absence of hemorrhage or xanthochromia in the spinal fluid. Once the diagnosis of peripheral embolism to an extremity is made, heparin therapy should be instituted without delay. Embolectomy is indicated unless the patient is moribund. The operation is usually done under local anesthesia using a Fogarty catheter. The Vascular Surgery Service should be notified at once, and arteriography is frequently performed prior to embolectomy. The mortality rate following such a procedure may approach 15%, with a limb salvage rate of about 95%, encouraging an aggressive surgical approach to this complication.

MYOCARDIAL RUPTURE

This is said to account for 10–15% of deaths due to acute MI. It usually occurs during the first week of the infarction and rarely in the first few hours. For some unknown reason it is more common in women. Systemic hypertension predisposes to it, and most patients die suddenly without premonitory symptoms. Occasionally patients complain of new or recurrent ischemic chest pain and present with cardiac tamponade. Although death usually occurs in a few minutes, some patients survive long enough to allow temporary relief of tamponade and transfer to the operating room where the defect can be closed.

SUGGESTED READING

Kossowsky, W. A., Epstein, P. J., and Levine, R. S. Post myocardial infarction syndrome; an early complication of acute myocardial infarction. *Chest* 63:35–40, 1973.

Sasahara, A. A., Sonnenblick, E. H., and Lesch, M. *Pulmonary Emboli.* New York: Grune & Stratton, 1974–1975.

Thompson, J. E. Acute peripheral arterial occlusions. *N. Engl. J. Med.* 290:950–952, 1974.

Biorck, G., Mogensen, L., Nyquist, O., Orinius, E., and Sjogren, A. Studies of myocardial rupture with cardiac tamponade in acute myocardial infarction. *Chest* 61: 4–13, 1972.

20

Modification of Myocardial Infarction Size

A variety of hemodynamic and pharmacologic interventions have been found to alter infarct size in experimental animal models of MI. Some of these interventions have been tested in patients with acute MI and preliminary results have been encouraging. It is still too early to recommend the routine use of most of them, but the existing experimental and clinical observations will be briefly reviewed. It is expected that future editions of this handbook will have something more definitive to say concerning reduction of infarct size as more extensive clinical trials are performed.

ALTERATION IN MYOCARDIAL OXYGEN DEMAND

Myocardial oxygen demand is a major factor in the survival of myocardial cells made critically ischemic (although still viable) during an acute infarction (see Chapter 1). Clearly, factors that increase myocardial oxygen consumption will adversely affect such cells and vice versa. Animal studies have demonstrated an adverse effect on infarct size, in nonfailing hearts, of tachycardia, isoproterenol, digitalis, and glucagon. In failing hearts, digitalis reduces infarct size, presumably by decreasing left ventricular dilatation and hence wall stress. Wall stress is one of the three major factors that determine myocardial oxygen consumption. The other two factors are heart rate and contractility (see Chapter 1). Beta adrenergic blocking agents reduce myocardial oxygen consumption and have been reported to reduce infarct size in both animals and man; major clinical trials of this class of pharmacologic agent are currently underway.

Balloon counterpulsation has been shown to reduce experimental infarct size partly by reducing left ventricular work, and hence myocardial oxygen demand, and partly by increasing myocardial blood flow (see below and Chapter 23).

Recent observations in humans suggest that arterial hypertension has a deleterious effect on infarct size and that treatment of such patients, with resultant normotension, can reduce infarct size (see Chapter 16).

It would be premature to recommend the routine use of beta blocking agents in acute MI. However, measures aimed at reducing tachycardia and left ventricular wall stress such as treatment of hypertension, volume depletion, heart failure, anxiety, and agitation are clearly indicated. The use of isoproterenol under any circumstance, and digitalis in nonfailing hearts, should be avoided.

IMPROVEMENT IN MYOCARDIAL BLOOD FLOW

As mentioned previously, counterpulsation has been shown to reduce experimental infarct size. Two mechanisms are operant here: decreased left ventricular oxygen demand and increased myocardial blood flow. Similarly, nitroglycerin has been shown to reduce infarct size in animals. The mechanism of nitroglycerin's beneficial effect is still contested but is probably secondary to decreased myocardial oxygen demand and increased myocardial blood flow. Nitroglycerin reduces left ventricular cavity size, and hence wall tension, by dilating large capacitance veins and pooling blood in the periphery. Increased myocardial blood flow occurs through collateral blood vessels because of the drug's direct vasodilating properties and because reduced left ventricular wall tension lessens systolic compression of collateral blood vessels. Coronary artery bypass surgery is capable of increasing myocardial blood flow but can rarely be performed rapidly enough (within four hours) following acute infarction to affect infarct size.

It is still too early to recommend routine counterpulsation and nitroglycerin therapy in acute infarction. However, encouraging results have been obtained in patients with acute MI and moderate left ventricular failure who were treated with external counterpulsation (see Chapter 23).

AUGMENTATION OF ENERGY SOURCES IN ISCHEMIC MYOCARDIUM

Increased levels of glucose, insulin, and potassium made available to anoxic heart preparations result in improved myocardial function, presumably secondary to increased intracellular levels of high energy phosphates which result from this "forced feeding" of myocardial cells.

The intravenous glucose-insulin-potassium regimen of Sodi-Pallares has been shown to reduce infarct size in animals. Clinical trials have produced conflicting results, and therefore one cannot advise the routine use of this program in the treatment of myocardial infarction. It seems reasonable, however, to provide such patients with a diet high in glucose and potassium (see Chapter 6).

IMPROVED DIFFUSION OF OXYGEN AND SUBSTRATES TO ISCHEMIC CELLS

Initial observations indicate that experimental and clinical infarct size can be reduced by means of intravenous hyaluronidase therapy, presumably because this agent increases diffusion through the extracellular space and hence may facilitate delivery of substrates to ischemic cells. Widespread use of this agent must await confirmation of these studies.

Recently, supplemental inspiratory oxygen has been shown to decrease infarct size in animals and man, presumably by increasing the diffusion of oxygen into ischemic areas of myocardium. These results support the current practice of administering supplemental inspiratory oxygen to patients with acute infarctions (see Chapter 9).

STABILIZATION OF AUTOLYTIC AND HETEROLYTIC PROCESSES IN SEVERELY ISCHEMIC MYOCARDIUM

The intravenous administration of pharmacological doses of corticosteroids has been shown to reduce experimental and clinical infarct size. The mechanisms of this effect are not totally clear but seem related to the drug's ability to stabilize lysosomal membranes and thus prevent the release of acidic hydrolases which may contribute to cellular damage. Routine use of these agents in MI must await further clinical studies, particularly in view of a recent study in which patients with acute MI received large doses of corticosteroids. Several patients in this study died secondary to myocardial free wall rupture.

SUGGESTED READING

Maroko, P. R., and Braunwald, E. Modification of myocardial infarction size after coronary occlusion. *Ann. Intern. Med.* 79:720–733, 1973.

Smith, E. R., Redwood, D. R., McCarron, W. E., and Epstein, S. E. Coronary artery occlusion in the conscious dog—effects of alterations in arterial pressure produced by nitroglycerin, hemorrhage, and alpha-adrenergic agonists on the degree of myocardial ischemia. *Circulation* 47:51–57, 1973.

Braunwald, E., and Maroko, P. R. The reduction of infarct size—an idea whose time (for testing) has come. *Circulation* 50:206–209, 1974.

Braunwald, E., and Maroko, P. R. Protection of the ischemic myocardium. *Hosp. Practice* 61–74, May, 1973.

Epstein, S. E., Kent, K. M., Goldstein, R. E., Boyer, J. S., and Redwood, D. R. Reduction of ischemic injury by nitroglycerin during acute myocardial infarction. *N. Engl. J. Med.* 292:29–35, 1975.

21

Anticoagulants in Acute Myocardial Infarction

The controversy concerning the use of anticoagulant therapy for acute MI began in 1938, prompted by a study that showed that intravenous heparin could prevent the formation of mural thrombi in dogs. The controversy that has surrounded this issue has been facilitated by defects in the structure of many of the studies on the use of anticoagulants in acute MI.

Anticoagulant therapy in acute MI primarily prevents venous thrombosis and pulmonary embolism (P.E.), although it may result in prevention of mural thrombus formation. The latter two complications account for approximately 6% of deaths from acute MI.

Deep vein thrombosis is not uncommon in patients with acute MI, occurring in as many as 37% of patients studied by the ^{125}I fibrinogen technique. Most of these patients never develop clinical thrombophlebitis or P.E. It has been established that patients with CHF and low-output syndrome, or patients confined to bed for a prolonged period of time, are at increased risk of developing venous thrombosis and P.E. It is in these patients that prophylactic anticoagulant therapy is most clearly indicated. The low-dose heparin regimen popularized by Kakkar and others is useful in such patients. This regimen is relatively free of bleeding complications and does not require laboratory monitoring. It is based on the observation that the formation of venous thrombosis depends upon the local accumulation of a critical concentration of activated factor X. Heparin enhances the action of the major inhibitor of activated factor X. The concentration of heparin required to inhibit the thrombus-forming reaction is considerably smaller than that necessary to prevent the process once thrombin has been formed.

Protocol

1. **The following categories of patients are candidates for low-dose heparin therapy: patients with sustained low-output syndrome or CHF; patients in whom prolonged bed rest is required. In some CCUs low-dose heparin is given routinely to all patients with acute MI.**
   a. **The usual dose of heparin is 5,000 units every eight to twelve hours given subcutaneously. Subcutaneous heparin should be administered in a small bolus injection into the abdominal wall or suprailiac crest fat employing a #25- or #26-gauge needle. The area should not be rubbed following the injection.**
2. **The following categories of patients are candidates for full systemic anticoagulation: patients with cardiogenic shock, arterial embolism (see Chapter 19), thrombophlebitis, or P.E. Protocol for administration of full doses of systemic heparin are to be found in Chapter 19. Many of these patients will require 2–3 months of oral anticoagulant (warfarin) therapy following discharge from the hospital. The decision to place the patient on oral anticoagulants must be individualized.**

SUGGESTED READING

Ebert, R. V. Use of anticoagulants in acute myocardial infarction. *Circulation* 45:903–910, 1972.

Gifford, R. H., and Feinstein, A. R. A critique of methodology in studies of anticoagulant therapy for acute myocardial infarction. *N. Engl. J. Med.* 280:351–357, 1969.

Modan, B., Shani, M., Schor, S., and Modan, M. Reduction of hospital mortality from acute myocardial infarction by anticoagulant therapy. *N. Engl. J. Med.* 292:1359–1362, 1975.

Tonascia, J., Gordis, L., and Schmerler, H. Retrospective evidence favoring use of anticoagulants for myocardial infarctions. *N. Engl. J. Med.* 292:1362–1366, 1975.

Electrical Cardioversion: Indications and Procedure

The history of the application of electrical energy to the heart began in the 18th century when the Danish scientist Abilgard delivered a direct-current shock to a chicken, resulting in lifelessness. Upon repetition of the shock, the bird took off and "eluded" further experimentation. Electrical cardioversion is now an essential feature of the coronary care unit in every hospital. The term *cardioversion* is generally used to mean the delivery of a specific and predetermined amount of electrical energy to the heart timed in such a way (synchronized) that the shock is delivered well away from the vulnerable period of the T wave of the ECG. Cardioversion may be performed electively or urgently with the patient lightly anesthetized. Defibrillation is the delivery of a large amount of electrical energy (usually 400 watt/sec) to a patient manifesting ventricular fibrillation. This latter procedure is performed without delay and without prior administration of an anesthetic agent, since the patient is usually unconscious. The procedure is considered safe and effective and is employed electively or urgently to terminate arrhythmias.

Electrical cardioversion is a safe and effective procedure when performed by experienced personnel. The overall success rate for termination of atrial and ventricular rhythm disturbances approaches 90%. Although the indications for its use in individual rhythm disturbances are discussed in Chapter 11 and basically include most non-sinus tachyarrhythmias in the setting of acute MI, the contraindications are of equal importance and are listed below:

1. Patients with atrial fibrillation with slow ventricular response associated with coronary artery disease

2. Patients with digitalis toxicity
3. Patients unable to maintain normal sinus rhythm (NSR) despite repeated cardioversions and antiarrhythmic drugs
4. Patients with the sick sinus syndrome who demonstrate both tachyarrhythmias and bradyarrhythmias (such patients should have a pacemaker in position if cardioversion is attempted, since severe bradycardia or asystole is not uncommon following this procedure)
5. Patients with long-standing (>5 years) atrial fibrillation with enlarged hearts
6. Patients with "lone" atrial fibrillation
7. Patients with atrial fibrillation due to untreated hyperthyroidism

The complication rate for this procedure is about 15%, not including minor skin burns and transient arrhythmias. The incidence of complications appears to be related to the energy level setting, being 6% at 150 watt/sec and 30% at 400 watt/sec. One rarely needs to set the initial energy level at 300 watt/sec or more except, of course, in cases of ventricular fibrillation. The following complications may occur:

1. Pulmonary or systemic emboli are seen in about 1.4% of cases. The incidence is similar to that following quinidine conversion, and systemic emboli are probably more likely to occur in patients with large left atria.
2. Increased serum enzymes (GOT, LDH, and CPK) occur in 10% of patients due to skeletal muscle trauma. The myocardial fraction of CPK (CPK-MB) is elevated in only a small percent of patients. In normal dogs it has been shown that countershock-induced myocardial necrosis is more likely to occur when the time interval between discharges is short and when smaller-sized paddle electrodes are used. During elective cardioversion, consecutive discharges should there-

fore be delivered at time intervals greater than three minutes.

3. Ventricular ectopy is more common at high-energy settings, even in the absence of digitalis and should be treated in the conventional manner (see Chapter 11).
4. Hypotension occurs in 3% of patients and may persist for several hours. The reason for this is not altogether clear, since recent echocardiographic data indicate that cardioversion promptly restores effective atrial contraction, decreases left atrial size, and results in substantial hemodynamic benefit.
5. Pulmonary edema and cardiomegaly occur in 3% of patients. It is seen once sinus rhythm has been restored, occurring 1–3 hours after the procedure. The mechanism is unknown.

It is clear that cardioversion is a safe and effective form of treatment for tachyarrhythmias seen in the setting of acute MI. Although the procedure is frequently used "electively" in the CCU, urgent termination of tachyarrhythmias is important because of the increase in myocardial oxygen consumption that occurs with these rhythm disturbances (see Chapter 11). The success and safety of the procedure is dependent on meticulous attention to the details of anesthesia, sedation, electrolytes, antiarrhythmic therapy, and anticoagulation.

Protocol

1. **The patient should be given a complete explanation with informed consent and the indications for the procedure should be documented in the chart.**
2. **The serum potassium level should be determined, and hypokalemia corrected if necessary.**
3. **A secure intravenous line should be in place and a 12-lead ECG obtained prior to cardioversion.**
4. **It is often advised that digitalis preparation be withheld for 24 hr before cardioversion to prevent ven-**

tricular arrhythmias. However, it is probably not necessary to discontinue digitalis therapy in patients with normal renal function and normal serum potassium who are receiving modest doses of the drug. Signs of digitalis toxicity generally preclude the use of cardioversion.

5. The nurse should prepare intravenous solutions of isoproterenol and lidocaine for immediate use, and syringes of atropine and of lidocaine should be readily available.
6. If the patient has been taking digitalis and this drug has not been withheld, a bolus of 75–100 mg of lidocaine IV is given prior to the procedure. Additionally, patients on digitalis should have the initial energy level set at 5 watt/sec. If this low-energy level results in frequent PVCs, the procedure should be abandoned.
7. The cardioversion equipment should be turned on ahead of time so "warm-up" can occur. The synchronizer (which allows the electrical discharge to occur on the R wave, away from the vulnerable period of the T wave) should always be tested before undertaking treatment by carefully examining the superimposed artifact on the ECG signal. Occasionally, especially in patients with anterior infarctions, there is not enough R wave voltage for the synchronizing unit to sense properly, and clinical judgment must be exercised whether to continue in the absence of synchronization. Some cardioversion units have a special switch that inverts the electrocardiographic tracing on the oscilloscope screen. This converts S waves to R waves and enables one to perform synchronized cardioversions in patients with poor or absent R waves.
8. The patient should be kept NPO for several hours prior to the procedure. Antiarrhythmic drugs such as quinidine are frequently given orally, however, 1–2 hr prior to the procedure (see Chapter 11) to maintain normal sinus rhythm (NSR) should cardioversion be successful. There is some controversy about this practice, although it seems reasonable that cardioversion would more likely be successful and NSR would be maintained if the patient already had antiarrhythmic drug therapy "on-board."

9. **Use of anticoagulants prior to cardioversion is controversial. However, most authors advise that patients with mitral stenosis or previous history of systemic embolism should be anticoagulated for at least several weeks prior to the procedure and for four weeks thereafter in an effort to prevent systemic embolism at the time of the procedure.**
10. **The paddles should be of adequate size and without dents or "pits" (caused by incorrectly testing the synchronizer by holding the paddles against each other). The preferred method in elective treatment is to put one paddle under the patient's back, just inferior to the left scapula and medial to the spine, and the other paddle over the precordium. The paddles should never be in contact with ECG leads. In more urgent circumstances, one paddle is placed at the base of the heart and the other at the apex. Good skin contact is necessary. A commercially available gel or dampened saline pads should be placed between the skin and the paddles to prevent skin burns. ECG cream should never be used for this purpose, since it carries too much resistance.**
11. **Equipment used in cardiac arrest situations (e.g., endotracheal tubes, etc.) must be readily available.**
12. **Amnesia is produced by repeated doses of 5 mg of diazepam given intravenously by the physician until the patient is lightly asleep. Many institutions prefer performing cardioversion under short-acting barbiturate anesthesia in the presence of an anesthesiologist.**
13. **Oxygen is provided by nasal prongs or mask. Lights should be dimmed and the room kept quiet to help alleviate the patient's anxiety and to improve the effect of the diazepam.**
14. **The energy is set at the appropriate level and the current is discharged; it should be kept in mind that in most synchronized units there is some slight time delay between "pressing the button" and actual cardioversion.**

SUGGESTED READING

Lown, B. Electrical reversion of cardiac arrhythmias. *Br. Heart J.* 29:469–489, 1967.

Resnekov, L., and McDonald, L. Appraisal of electrocardioversion in treatment of dysrhythmias. *Br. Heart J.* 30:786–811, 1968.

Resnekov, L. Present status of electroversion in the management of cardiac dysrhythmias. *Circulation* 47:1356–1363, 1973.

Counterpulsation in Patients with Myocardial Infarction or Unstable Angina: Indications and Procedure

Counterpulsation is a technique whereby the volume of blood in the aorta is transiently increased during diastole by means of a mechanical device. This sudden increase in aortic diastolic volume results in an increase in aortic diastolic pressure.

The majority of left ventricular coronary blood flow occurs during diastole. Hence, increased aortic diastolic blood pressure results in a greater perfusion pressure for the coronary bed during diastole. This increased perfusion forces more blood through a stenotic coronary arterial system and thus increases myocardial blood flow in patients with coronary artery disease. It is obvious that increased myocardial blood flow benefits the patient with critical myocardial ischemia.

Two forms of counterpulsation are commonly in use. Internal or balloon counterpulsation requires the placement of an elongated, sausage-shaped balloon in the descending aorta. The balloon is inserted through a tubular, Dacron graft side arm sewn onto the patient's femoral artery. The balloon, triggered by the ECG, is rapidly inflated with CO_2 or helium during cardiac diastole, thus transiently increasing aortic volume and pressure. At the very onset of systole, the balloon is rapidly deflated, creating a minor vacuum in the aorta that has the effect of sucking blood out of the left ventricle and hence reducing cardiac work.

External counterpulsation involves surrounding the patient's lower extremities (from ankle to upper thigh) with a plastic water mattress. The water pressure within this mattress is increased to 150–200 mm Hg during cardiac diastole. External compression of the legs forces arterial blood back into the aorta and venous blood forward into the vena cava. Thus, diastolic aortic and vena caval volume and pressure increase, resulting in simultaneous increases in ventricular filling and myocardial blood flow.

Both forms of counterpulsation are effective in supporting the circulation of animals with experimental cardiogenic shock and of patients with that clinical entity. Moreover, there is evidence that counterpulsation reduces experimental infarct size in animals and morbidity and mortality in patients with MI and moderate degrees of left ventricular failure (see Chapter 20). It would appear that internal or balloon counterpulsation affords greater hemodynamic support than external counterpulsation, although the differences between the two methods are not great.

Current indications for counterpulsation include: (1) cardiogenic shock (see Chapter 15) secondary to MI or following cardiac surgery; (2) highly unstable angina pectoris (see Chapter 17); and (3) severe left ventricular failure with or without acute mitral regurgitation or ventricular septal rupture (see Chapter 14). The combination of counterpulsation and afterload reduction with nitroprusside (see Chapter 13) has been shown to be particularly effective in selected patients with severe left ventricular failure. Counterpulsation is contraindicated in patients with aortic dissection, large aortic aneurysms, and aortic regurgitation.

The application and correct use of counterpulsation devices requires some training. It should be performed by a knowledgeable team who can be rapidly mobilized at any time. The insertion of the aortic balloon is usually performed by a thoracic or vascular surgeon. In the case of a patient felt to be a candidate for counterpulsation, Cardiology and Cardiac Surgery should be consulted. It is particularly important to consult Cardiac Surgery in such cases because patients who require counterpulsation rarely survive for more than a few days or weeks without a definitive surgical procedure (e.g., coronary artery bypass, mitral valve replacement, closure of ventricular septal defect, or aneurysmectomy). (See Chapter 25.)

SUGGESTED READING

Resnekov, L. Mechanical assistance for the failing ventricle. *Mod. Concepts Cardiovasc. Dis.* 43:81–85, 1974.

Scheidt, S., et al. Intra-aortic balloon counterpulsation in cardiogenic shock: report of a co-operative clinical trial. *N. Engl. J. Med.* 288:979–984, 1973.

Soroff, H. S., Cloutier, C. T., Birtwell, W. C., Begley, L. A., and Messer, J. V. External counterpulsation—measurement of cardiogenic shock after myocardial infarction. *J.A.M.A.* 229:1441–1450, 1974.

Amsterdam, E. A., Messer, J. V., Willerson, J. W., Loeb, H. S., Criley, M., Banas, J., and Mason, D. T. Clinical assessment of external pressure circulatory assist in acute myocardial infarction. Abstract, *Am. J. Cardiol.* 37:116, 1976.

24

Flow-directed Catheter Insertion, Arterial Line Insertion, and Interpretation of Data

Recently, hemodynamic monitoring has come to play a crucial role in the management of critically ill patients with acute MI. Hemodynamic measurements made in patients soon after hospitalization for acute MI usually demonstrate elevated left ventricular end-diastolic pressures (LVEDP). It has generally been accepted that this increase in LVEDP shortly after acute MI is usually due to an increase in stiffness (decreased compliance) of the left ventricle but may also result from an increase in left ventricular end-diastolic volume.

Elevations of LVEDP are transmitted to the left atrium and thence to the pulmonary capillaries. (Normal LVEDP = 3–10 mm Hg; normal pulmonary capillary wedge pressure = 1–10 mm Hg.) Marked elevation of LVEDP (and hence PCW) can result in interstitial and eventually alveolar pulmonary edema (at wedge pressures >25 mm Hg). Recent clinical observations have documented that Starling's law operates in patients with acute MI: increases in LVEDP result in increases in cardiac output until a plateau is reached. Pulmonary artery catheterization via a flow-directed balloon catheter in patients with acute MI allows one to estimate a Starling curve for each patient catheterized. Cardiac output is determined by the Fick principle, by dye, or thermal indicator dilution curves while LVEDP is gauged from the PCW. A PCW of 15–18 mm Hg results in optimal cardiac output in most patients with acute MI.

Although an attempt should be made to identify A, C, and V waves in the PCW position, this is not always possible. Large, peaked V waves should alert one to the possibility of acute mitral regurgitation (see

Chapter 14). In the CCU the mean PCW pressure (integrated electrically by the equipment) is conventionally recorded. One should remember that there are other causes of elevated PCW besides left ventricular dysfunction (e.g., mitral stenosis). Patients with chronic lung disease should have normal PCW unless there is associated left ventricular disease. However, patients with COPD tend to have marked respiratory variation in their PCW tracings, and the highest level during expiration and the lowest level during inspiration should be obtained and these values averaged.

The following are the indications for insertion of arterial lines and/or pulmonary artery catheters. Clearly, each patient should be considered individually before the decision for invasive monitoring is made.

1. Cardiogenic shock or hypotension (see Chapter 15).
2. Severe left ventricular failure with pulmonary edema, mitral regurgitation, and/or ventricular septal rupture (see Chapters 13 and 14).
3. Significant systemic hypertension complicating acute myocardial infarction (see Chapter 16).
4. Significant and persistent sinus tachycardia (120–150 beats/min). Such patients are frequently found to have low filling pressures; the heart rate may be lowered in such patients by adequate volume expansion (see Chapters 11 and 13).

Protocol

1. **Insertion of the flow-directed catheter can be accomplished percutaneously through the right femoral vein using the same modified Seldinger technique as described for pacemakers (see Chapter 12). Many institutions prefer to insert these catheters via antecubital vein "cut-down" or percutaneous subclavian routes.**
2. **The procedure should be discussed with the patient or**

next of kin and a note placed in the patient's chart explaining the indications.

3. It is important that the pressure equipment be calibrated, flushed, and "ready to go" before the catheter is introduced into the pulmonary artery.
4. The larger 7 French catheter is preferred because of the ease of withdrawing blood samples for oxygen saturation determination.
5. Although fluoroscopy is not necessary when introducing this catheter into the pulmonary artery (PA) and pulmonary capillary wedge (PCW) positions, the equipment should be ready on standby should it be needed. Appropriate catheter position is easily checked with fluoroscopy.
6. It is important to test the integrity of the balloon before introducing it into the vein by inflating it underwater with 0.8 cc of air with a 1 ml plastic syringe.
7. Once introduced into the vein, the catheter should be advanced to the right atrium, which is usually a distance of about 35 cm if the arm or leg is used (markers are placed at 10 cm distances along the shaft of the catheter). When the catheter tip is in the thorax, a cough will produce marked deflections in the pressure tracing.
8. Once the tip of the catheter is in the thorax, 0.8 to 1.5 cc of air (in the 7 French catheter) is introduced into the balloon.
9. The catheter is then gently advanced through the right atrium, right ventricle (RV), and PA to the PCW position, each chamber position being documented by the characteristic pressure tracing.
10. After passage of the catheter into the PCW position, the balloon should be deflated. The time period during which the wedge pressure is recorded must be kept to a minimum in order to lessen the stress on the wall of the pulmonary artery and to prevent pulmonary infarction. This is especially important in patients with chronic pulmonary arterial hypertension. The catheter, when not measuring PCW, should rest in the PA, verified by a PA pressure tracing.
11. When inflating the balloon to record PCW, one should

slowly add air until the pressure tracing changes from the PA to the PCW configuration. If considerably less air is needed to obtain a PCW than that recommended on the shaft of the catheter, one can assume that the catheter has migrated too far into the wedge position, and it should be gradually pulled back into a position where full or near-full balloon inflation volume is needed to record wedge pressure. Remember that inflation must be performed slowly and stopped when the change from PA to PCW is noted. Should the catheter tip migrate to the PCW position for prolonged periods of time, pulmonary infarction may be induced. Frequent monitoring of the catheter tip is therefore necessary. If fluoroscopy is not used, a chest x-ray should be performed following the procedure to check the catheter position. PAW and pulmonary artery end-diastolic pressures are usually within a few mm Hg of each other.

12. Fluid should not be used to inflate the balloon, since it may be irretrievable. To prevent unintentional injection of fluids, it is recommended that the inflation syringe be kept constantly attached to the balloon lumen.
13. A constant infusion through the catheter lumen should be maintained at all times, and small amounts of heparin (10,000 u/1,000 cc of infusate) should be added to this solution.
14. The balloon should be deflated when the catheter is removed.
15. Cardiac index by the Fick principle is determined as follows:
    a. Obtain simultaneous or near-simultaneous pulmonary arterial and systemic arterial blood samples in heparinized syringes for blood gas analysis.
    b. Calculate the oxygen content of these samples as described in the Protocol in Chapter 14 (step 3).
    c. Determine the patient's total body oxygen consumption with a Douglas bag and the help of the Catheterization Laboratory or assume 125 cc/min/M^2.
    d. Calculate cardiac index from the following formula:

Cardiac index (L/min/M²)

$$= \frac{\text{oxygen consumption index or assume 125 cc/min/M}^2}{\text{systemic arterial } O_2 \text{ content} - \text{pulmonary arterial } O_2 \text{ content}}$$

e. **Normal cardiac index is generally ≥2.8 L/min/M². Normal pulmonary arterial oxygen saturation is 75%, and normal systemic arterial oxygen saturation is 95%.**

The technique for systemic arterial pressure monitoring varies. Most CCUs employ the radial, brachial, or femoral arteries. The last two routes are preferred because the catheter tip is closest to the central aorta. Systemic arterial lines allow one to obtain frequent recordings of systemic blood pressure and blood samples for arterial blood gas analysis.

A mean systemic arterial pressure of 70 mm Hg is required to maintain adequate glomerular filtration. A peak systolic pressure of 90 mm Hg may be appropriate for a given patient, provided he shows no clinical signs of hypoperfusion. The blood pressure determined by cuff may underestimate the actual intra-arterial pressure by 10 mm Hg or more.

Protocol

1. **Percutaneous insertion of small Teflon catheters into the radial, brachial, or femoral arteries can usually be accomplished by means of the Seldinger technique. This technique has been previously described for venous catheterization (see Chapter 12). Several differences should be noted between the venous and arterial Seldinger techniques:**
   a. **In the arterial Seldinger technique, the Seldinger needle is aimed directly at the arterial pulsation.**
   b. **No syringe is placed on the Seldinger needle during withdrawal. A large (1–2 in. arc) pulsating stream of blood emerges from the end of the needle when its tip is completely within the lumen of the artery.**
   c. **No attempt should be made to thread the guide wire through the Seldinger needle unless a pulsating**

stream of blood is emerging from the end of the needle.

2. **Once the Teflon catheter is inserted over the guide wire and into the artery, it should be well secured to prevent accidental dislodgment.**
3. **Peripheral pulses (beyond a brachial or femoral arterial catheterization) should be monitored daily, and the catheter withdrawn if signs of arterial insufficiency develop.**
4. **The arterial line should be continuously flushed by means of a one-way valve and a pressurized plastic bag containing a heparinized (10,000 u/1,000 cc 5% D/W) infusate.**

SUGGESTED READING

Russell, R. O., Rackley, C. E., Pombo, J., Hunt, D., Potanin, C., and Dodge, H. T. Effects of increasing left ventricular filling pressure in patients with acute myocardial infarction. *J. Clin. Invest.* 49:1539–1550, 1970.

Falicov, R. E., and Resnekov, L. Relationship of the pulmonary artery end-diastolic pressure to the left ventricular end-diastolic and mean filling pressures in patients with and without left ventricular dysfunction. *Circulation* 42:65–78, 1970.

Swan, H. J. C., Ganz, W., Forrester, J., Marcus, H., Diamond, G., and Chonette, D. Catheterization of the heart in man with the use of a flow-directed balloon-tipped catheter. *N. Engl. J. Med.* 283:447–451, 1970.

Gardner, R. M., Schwartz, R., Wong, H. C., and Burk, J. P. Percutaneous indwelling radial-artery catheters for monitoring cardiovascular function—prospective study of the risk of thrombus and infection. *N. Engl. J. Med.* 290:1227–1231, 1974.

Cardiac Catheterization and Cardiac Surgery

Urgent or emergency cardiac catheterization and cardiac surgery are desperate measures in a patient with an acute MI. Both procedures are associated with considerably higher risk in patients with acute infarction as compared to individuals with remote infarcts (at least 2–3 months post infarction). However, in an occasional critically ill patient cardiac surgery can be lifesaving. Counterpulsation devices (see Chapter 23) enable the physician to stabilize many of these critically ill individuals and thus gain time for the consideration of cardiac catheterization and surgery.

Patients in the following diagnostic categories may be candidates for urgent or emergency catheterization and surgery. Counterpulsation is usually employed before, during, and after catheterization in such patients. In addition, counterpulsation is frequently required for several days (occasionally longer) following cardiac surgery.

1. Cardiogenic shock (see Chapter 15). An occasional patient with cardiogenic shock can be salvaged by means of coronary artery bypass. Some surgeons perform an associated infarctectomy. Unless a mechanical deficit such as mitral regurgitation or ventricular septal rupture can be corrected (see item 3 below), few patients survive.
2. Unstable angina pectoris refractory to medical management following infarction (see Chapter 18) or in the absence of infarction (see Chapter 17). These two groups include patients who continue to have angina with minimal or no exertion despite hospitalization on optimal medical regimens. Surgery for such patients usually consists of coronary bypass with occasional infarctectomy and/or aneurysmectomy in postinfarction pa-

tients. Mortality is inversely proportional to the adequacy of left ventricular function: the more normal the left ventricular function, the lower the mortality.

Many of the patients in this category will be on significant doses of propranolol, although many surgeons are reluctant to have patients come to cardiopulmonary bypass while on this therapy. On the other hand, rapid cessation of propranolol therapy has precipitated MI in some patients. Consequently, it is strongly advised that if propranolol is to be discontinued before surgery, it be done gradually by tapering the dosage over several days or more. It is usually necessary to hospitalize such patients, increase their sedation and nitrates, and observe them closely. Many cardiologists feel that propranolol can be safely continued right up to the time of surgery. Should propranolol be discontinued, any increase in anginal frequency or intensity should result in the reinitiation of propranolol therapy.

3. Severe left ventricular failure with acute mitral regurgitation or ventricular septal rupture (see Chapters 13 and 14). Appropriate surgical procedures in selected patients include various combinations of coronary bypass grafting, mitral valve replacement, and ventricular septal repair.
4. Recurrent, life-threatening ventricular arrhythmias (e.g., VT, VF) refractory to medical therapy. Selected patients with this devastating problem have responded to coronary artery bypass grafting, usually in combination with infarctectomy and/or aneurysmectomy.

SUGGESTED READING

Mundth, E. D., and Austen, W. G. Surgical measures for coronary heart disease. *N. Engl. J. Med.* 293:13–19, 75–80, 124–130, 1975.

Keon, W. J., Bedard, P., Kanakaiahnavava, R. S., Akyurekli, Y., Nino, A., and Berkman, F. Experience with emergency aortocoronary bypass grafts in the presence of acute myocardial infarction. *Circulation* (Suppl. III) 47, 48:III–151, III–155, 1973.

26

Cardiac Rehabilitation and Follow-up of Patients after Discharge from the Hospital

Rehabilitation is defined as a process that begins with the onset of an injury and the object of which is to restore and maintain the individual's physiological, social, and vocational status. When the patient has recovered from the initial trauma associated with acute MI and has been transferred to the Intermediate Cardiac Unit, the pathophysiology and significance of what has happened should be explained in detail to the patient and his/her family. Questions about the plan of management, medications, prognosis, and resumption of sexual and job activity should be considered at that time. Pamphlets and cassette tape/movies are frequently helpful in this regard. Nursing personnel should ideally have specialized training in this area as well, since they usually spend far more time with the patient than does the physician. It is particularly important that risk factors be identified and corrected. The serum lipid levels and carbohydrate metabolism do not usually return to preinfarction levels until about three weeks after acute MI (i.e., cholesterol and triglyceride are usually spuriously low following acute MI, while blood glucose is sometimes "falsely elevated"). Depending upon how well the patient has done during the ambulation period prior to discharge, most patients can return to work 6–8 weeks after their infarction. Patients should not be allowed to engage in vigorous physical activity or heavy lifting while at home. It is frequently helpful to give each patient a handout sheet which specifically defines what he/she can and cannot do after discharge.

Most patients are taught to take their pulse rate, and they are instructed not to engage in activity that produces a heart rate greater than 120 beats/min. Around the time of the first visit to the doctor following discharge from the hospital (about 3–4 weeks after acute MI), a submaximal exercise test is performed to assess the patient's exercise tolerance and stability of rhythm during exercise. During this test the heart rate is not allowed to exceed 120 beats/min. The test is roughly equivalent to climbing two flights of stairs or walking 2,500 feet. If this test is satisfactory, the patient is given a gradual walking exercise program and is allowed to resume sexual activity. By the sixth week after infarction most patients are able to walk a distance of one-half mile and to return to work. The patient is instructed to seek immediate medical attention should he develop complications such as recurrent chest pain. The patient should also avoid those things that provoke angina pectoris, and the prophylactic use of nitroglycerin is encouraged.

The patient then returns to the clinic about eight weeks after infarction and by now should be walking about one mile per day without difficulty. A second exercise test is then performed, this time allowing the patient to achieve 70% of maximal predicted heart rate (about 150 beats/min for most people) provided no difficulties (e.g., arrhythmias, angina) are encountered. If the patient can perform this level of exercise without angina or serious arrhythmias, he/she may enter into a medically supervised exercise program, provided there are no complicating factors (such as arrhythmias, cardiomegaly, mitral regurgitation, and conduction disturbances). This is clearly an important decision which must be made individually after careful evaluation. At no time should the patient be encouraged to engage in jogging or any other exercise program without careful preliminary evaluation and medical supervision of the exercise program.

Not all patients can be entered into a cardiac rehabilitation program, and not all patients desire this kind of program. All patients should, however, be encouraged to lead an active lifestyle once they have successfully convalesced from their acute MI. Without a careful assessment of exercise tolerance and cardiac rhythm in the postinfarction period, however, it is impossible to prescribe a rational program of rehabilitation. Objective data including Holter monitoring and graded exercise tests are helpful in developing this prescription.

Protocol

1. Rehabilitation begins once the patient has been discharged from the CCU. Patient education should be offered during the second week of convalescence.

2. At discharge the patient should be carefully instructed concerning medicines and activities. Moderate activity around the house is allowed at this time (but no isometric exercises such as lifting).

a. The patient should be given sublingual nitroglycerin tablets at this time and he/she should be instructed in their use.

3. Approximately 1–2 weeks after discharge the patient undergoes a submaximal treadmill test (maximal heart rate = 120 beats/min). If this is performed without angina, ST segment change, or arrhythmia, the patient is allowed to walk ¼–½ mile/day and to resume sexual activity.

a. If angina, ST segment change, or arrhythmia occur, further pharmacologic intervention is probably indicated (e.g., nitrates, propranolol, digoxin, diuretics—depending upon the individual patient and his/her status).

b. Patients with an abnormal treadmill response should not increase their activity level until improvement has occurred as documented by a subsequent treadmill test or Holter monitor tape.

4. At 6 weeks after discharge the patient walks ½ mile/day comfortably and may return to work.

5. At 8 weeks after discharge the patient walks 1 mile/day comfortably and another treadmill exercise test is performed (to 70% predicted maximal heart rate or about 150 beats/min).

a. If this treadmill test is performed without incident, the patient is a candidate for a medically supervised exercise program (e.g., jogging, exercises, etc.).

SUGGESTED READING

Fox, S. M., Naughton, J. P., and Gorman, P. A. Physical activity and cardiovascular health. The exercise prescription: intensity and duration. *Mod. Concepts Cardiovasc. Dis.* 41:21–24, 1972.

Fox, S. M., Naughton, J. P., Gorman, P. A. Physical activity and cardiovascular health. The exercise prescription: frequency and type of activity. *Mod. Concepts Cardiovasc. Dis.* 41:25–30, 1972.

Appendix I

Indications, Routes, and Doses of Commonly Employed Medications

A. Guide for Rapid Administration of Antiarrhythmic Drugs (Intravenous Route)

Drug	Dose	Therapeutic Plasma Level (μg/ml)	Side effects	Comment
Lidocaine	100 mg IV bolus over several minutes followed by 2–4 mg/min constant infusion. 75 mg IV bolus for patients with pulmonary edema and 50 mg bolus for patients in shock.	1.4–6.0	Focal seizures, grand mal seizures, respiratory arrest, dizziness, heart block (usually associated with preexisting abnormal His-Purkinje conduction), sinoatrial arrest	Significant reduction in dose in patients with heart failure, moderate reduction in dose in patients with hepatic disease; no oral form available; no significant myocardial depression; toxicity usually seen at high plasma levels; toxicity at low plasma levels may be caused by metabolites.

Table A (Continued)

Drug	Dose	Therapeutic Plasma Level (μg/ml)	Side effects	Comment
Procainamide	100 mg IV slowly (50 mg/min) every 5 min (or more often in life-threatening situations) up to 1,000 mg	4–8	Hypotension, prolonged AV and His-Purkinje conduction	Myocardial toxicity usually only at high plasma levels or after rapid administration
Propranolol	1 mg/min IV up to 10 mg	40–85 (ng/ml)	Hypotension, bradycardia, prolonged AV conduction and heart block, myocardial depression, bronchospasm	Should probably not be considered in the presence of heart failure; many of the side effects reversed by large doses of isoproterenol
Diphenylhydantoin	50–100 mg IV slowly (50 mg/min) every 5 min up to 1,000 mg. Additional 500 mg on following day	10–18	Hypotension, 1:1 conduction in atrial flutter, respiratory arrest, idioventricular rhythm, ventricular fibrillation, asystole	Administration IM provides erratic blood levels; toxicity usually seen only after rapid administration
Atropine	0.6–1.0 mg IV as a rapid bolus	–	Sinus tachycardia, glaucomic crisis, urinary retention, psychosis	Occasionally precipitates paradoxical slowing of heart rate or ventricular tachycardia

B. Guide to Rapid Administration of Drugs Employed in the Treatment of Heart Failure or Shock (Intravenous Route)

Drug	Dose	Therapeutic Plasma Level (μg/ml)	Side effects	Comments
Digoxin	0.25 mg IV q8h for two days and then 0.25 mg q.d.	1.0–2.0 (ng/ml)	GI toxicity, cardiac arrhythmias, AV conduction disturbances, insomnia, visual disturbances	May be given orally with the same dose and rate of administration; should not be given intramuscularly
Furosemide	20–40 mg IV (or more) as needed	–	Ototoxicity, dehydration	Ethacrynic acid is an acceptable alternative
Nitroprusside	15–200 μg/min by gradually increasing a continuous IV infusion	–	Hypotension, anemia, hypothyroidism	Direct arterial pressure monitoring essential
Dopamine	Start with 2–5 μg/kg/min; increase to maximum of 50 μg/kg/min	–	Cardiac arrhythmias, gangrene of extremities	Direct arterial pressure monitoring advised
Norepinephrine	2–8 μg/min; start with low dose and increase gradually every 3–4 min	–	Cardiac arrhythmias, acute tubular necrosis, gangrene of extremities	Direct arterial pressure monitoring advised; beware of subcutaneous injection of infusate

C. Guide for Long-term Oral Administration of Antiarrhythmic Drugs

Drug	Usual Total Daily Dose	Frequency of Administration	Therapeutic Plasma Level (μg/ml)	Half-life (hr)	Side effects	Comments
Propranolol	80–320 mg	Every 6 hours	40–85 (ng/ml)	3–4.6	Myocardial depression, prolonged AV conduction and heart block, bradycardia, bronchospasm, fatigue, depression, peripheral vascular insufficiency, hyperglycemia, hypoglycemia, alopecia, gastric distention	Active metabolites may play a role in clinical effect; dose chosen empirically; should be tapered slowly in patients with angina; caution needed in patients with cardiac function dependent on sympathetic tone
Procainamide	2–6 g	Every 3–4 hours	4–8	3–4	Nausea, vomiting, agranulocytosis, lupuslike syndrome, myocardial depression, prolonged AV and His-Purkinje conduction	Toxic myocardial effect, usually only at toxic plasma levels; half-life markedly prolonged in renal failure or alkaline urine

Diphenylhydantoin	300–400 mg	Once daily	10–18	22	Nystagmus, ataxia, lethargy, nausea, vertigo, rashes, pseudolymphoma, megaloblastic anemia, peripheral neuropathy, hyperglycemia, seizures	Half-life higher at higher doses; rate of metabolism affected by many drugs; clinically significant decrease in plasma binding in azotemia and hypoproteinemia; should initiate therapy with 1.0 g loading dose
Quinidine	1.0–2.4 g	Every 6 hours	2.3–5.0 (using double extraction; higher for precipitation assay)	7	Hypotension, nausea, vomiting, diarrhea, tinnitus, vertigo, prolonged His-Purkinje conduction, rash, fever, thrombocytopenia, hepatic dysfunction, hemolytic anemia, ventricular arrhythmias	Minor gastrointestinal side effects controlled with symptomatic therapy; clinically significant decrease in plasma binding in hypoproteinemia and hepatic disease; myocardial toxicity usually only at toxic plasma levels; accumulation of metabolites in renal disease

Appendix II

Calculation of Peel and Norris Prognostic Indices

A. Peel Index: Using the table below, select one score from each of the six categories. Total the six numbers and estimate the associated mortality from the Peel Mortality Table.

1. Age and sex

MEN	54 or under	0	WOMEN	64 or under	2
	55–59	1		65 or more	3
	60–64	2			
	65 or more	3			

2. Previous history of coronary disease

Previous myocardial infarction	6
Other cardiovascular disease or history of dyspnea on exertion	3
Previous angina	1
No cardiovascular disease	0

3. Shock

Absent	0
Mild and transient	1
Moderate (present on admission but resolving with rest and sedation)	5
Severe and persistent	7

4. Left ventricular failure

Absent	0
Basilar rales	1
Any of the following: dyspnea at rest, pulmonary edema, orthopnea, S_3, hepatomegaly, elevated jugular venous pressure, peripheral edema	4

5. ECG

Normal QRS (ST-T changes only)	1
QR complexes	3
QS complexes or bundle-branch block	4

6. Rhythm

NSR	0
Any of the following: atrial fibrillation or flutter, PAT, frequent PVCs, nodal rhythm, heart block	4

Peel Mortality Table

Score:	1–8	9–12	13–16	17–20	21–28
Mortality:	2.5%	12.5%	23.7%	53.4%	88.5%

B. Norris Index: The X numerical weightings are multiplied by the corresponding Y number. Select only one score from each of the six areas. The index is constructed by adding together the six XY products. Mortality is estimated from the Norris Mortality Table.

Factor	*X*	*Y*
1. Age (yr)		
<50	0.2	
50–59	0.4	
60–69	0.6	3.9
70–79	0.8	
80–89	1.0	
2. Position of infarct		
Anterior transmural	1.0	
Left bundle-branch block	1.0	
Inferior and/or posterior transmural	0.7	2.8
Anterior subendocardial	0.3	
Inferior and/or posterior subendocardial	0.3	
3. Admission systolic blood pressure (mm Hg)		
<55	1.0	
55–64	0.7	
65–74	0.6	
75–84	0.5	
85–94	0.4	10.0
95–104	0.3	
105–114	0.2	
115–124	0.1	
>125	0.0	
4. Heart size (portable AP upright x-ray taken at 5 feet)		
Normal	0.0	
Doubtfully enlarged	0.5	1.5
Definitely enlarged	1.0	
5. Lung fields (portable AP upright x-ray taken at 5 feet)		
Normal	0.0	
Venous congestion	0.3	
Interstitial edema	0.6	3.3
Pulmonary edema	1.0	
6. Previous history of angina and/or infarction		
No ischemia	0.0	
Previous angina or infarction	1.0	

Norris Mortality Table

Score:	<4	4–5	6–7	8–9	10–11	12
Mortality:	3%	8%	22%	40%	65%	78%

Appendix III

Nomogram for Calculating Body Surface Area (BSA) from Height and Weight (in M²)

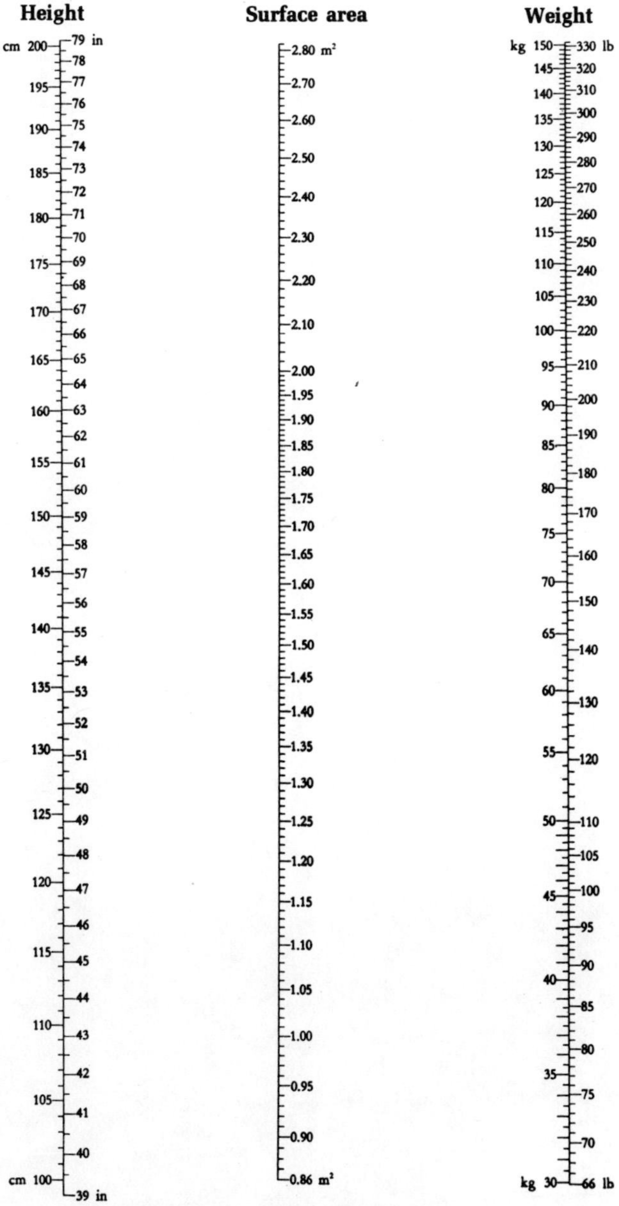

Index